GYNAECOLOGY
&
OBSTETRIC
THERAPEUTICS

BY
Dr. SHRIKANT KULKARNI
G.C.E.H. , DEAN,
Homoeopathic Medical College. Solapur.
CHIEF MEDICAL OFFICER,
Homoeopathic Hospital. Solapur.
Honorary Homoeopathic Physician to-
* Central Railway. Solapur, * Solapur Telephones, * Police Headquarters.

B. JAIN PUBLISHERS PVT. LTD.
An ISO 9001 : 2000 Certified Company
USA — EUROPE — INDIA

GYNAECOLOGY
&
OBSTETRIC
THERAPEUTICS

BY

DR SHRIKANT KULKARNI

G.C.E.H., DEAN

Homoeopathic Medical College, Solapur

CHIEF MEDICAL OFFICER,

Homoeopathic Hospital, Solapur

Honorary Homoeopathic Physician to-

* Central Railway, Solapur, * Solapur Telephones, * Police Headquarters.

B. JAIN PUBLISHERS PVT. LTD.

AN ISO 9001: 2000 CERTIFIED COMPANY

USA — EUROPE — INDIA

GYNAECOLOGY & OBSTETRIC THERAPEUTICS

First Edition: 1994
Reprint Edition: 1995, 1997, 2001, 2003, 2004, 2005, 2006, 2008

Published by Kuldeep Jain for
B. JAIN PUBLISHERS (P) LTD.
An ISO 9001 : 2000 Certified Company
1921/10, Chuna Mandi, Paharganj, New Delhi 110 055 (INDIA)
Tel.: +91-11-2358 0800, 2358 1100, 2358 1300, 2358 3100
Fax: +91-11-2358 0471 • *Email:* info@bjain.com
Website: **www.bjainbooks.com**

Printed in India
B.B Press, Noida

ISBN: 978-81-319-0106-9

DEDICATED

TO MY FATHER,

DADA,

WHO IS SO FOND OF READING.

PREFACE

A homoeopathic physician takes the complete case, the relevant history, the signs and symptoms and from this data he selects the similimum for a given case. How simple it looks on the paper! Indeed it is a very difficult task at the bedside of the patient, to find out or to select true similimum, the curative remedy for a particular case. To achieve this and to get success in prescribing the correct remedy deep knowledge of Homoeopathic Materia Medica and clear understanding of Organon of Medicine are of utmost necessity.

After inventing the "Therapeutic Law of Cure", Dr. Hahnemann laid down certain principles and rules for selecting and prescribing homoeopathic medicines to the patient. We are supposed to observe these laws during our practice; while selecting the remedy. Homoeopathic Materia Medica as a subject is very vast to memorise; the various drugs and their guiding symptoms, along with their modalities are beyond the capacity of human brain. We have not only to remember the remedy but also to implement logical sense while selecting the same.

We consider the patient as a whole. For that, while prescribing the medicine for a given case it is understood that we have considered particular symptoms of the disease for which patient has come to the hospital. General symptoms and concomitant symptoms give us the portrait of the disease. We consider this totality of symptoms to select the correct and most similar remedy.

Keeping this in mind I have tried to explain few gynaecological and obstetrical conditions in this book. In our day-to-day practice we do come across such cases frequently. I have described particular, characteristic, and striking symptom along with mental symptoms. Modalities are mentioned at the bottom.

As homoeopathy believes in individualisation, it is not correct to think of a specific drug for a specific condition. But still, I feel, this book would be helpful to the busy practitioners and to my students of final year DHMS/BHMS courses as readymade material. The student will get an idea of how to describe a particular drug in the therapeutics answer paper and my colleagues will be able to select the remedy for their patient within a short time.

My beloved teacher Dr. Mrs. Manjiri Chitale, has given me her full co-operation, expertise and every opportunity to study the cases in her consulting room, in wards and in the labour room. Her effective teaching, experience and skilled techniques made me to think on the subject from a different angle.

I shall be very happy and I shall consider it the best return for my efforts put in this book if it proves useful for my students and for the physicians.

"MAHASHIVARATRI"
19th February, 1994.

SHRIKANT M KULKARNI
312, SOUTH SADAR BAZAR,
CAMP, SOLAPUR-413003.
(MAHARASHTRA)

CONTENTS

Chapter - V

DISEASES OF UTERUS

Chapter - VI

DISEASES OF BREAST

Chapter - VII

GENERAL CONDITIONS

Chapter - VIII

OBSTETRICS THERAPEUTICS

CHAPTER 1

MENSTRUAL DISORDERS

TOPIC 1

LEUCORRHOEA

1.1.1 ALUMINA

There are three main reasons why Alumina patient suffers from leucorrhoea. The first and very important reason is recurrent infections, both systemic and local. Patient has abnormal craving for charcoal, chalk, mud etc. Secondly there is lack of exercise and the third important reason is anaemia. Uncleanliness during the period of menstruation causes leucorrhoea. Discharges are acrid, profuse, transparent and ropy; with burning sensation in genitalia. This burning sensation is relieved by washing the parts with cold water. Yellowish mucus runs through medial aspects of thighs down to heels; with scanty, delayed and pale menses. Patient is exhausted after menses and leucorrhoea. Leucorrhoea with constipation and anaemia.

Dryness of all the mucous membranes, the skin and the vagina. Patient is chilly. Sluggish functions, heaviness, numbness and staggering. Lack of vital heat and the peculiar constipation are the characteristic symptoms of Alumina. Stitching and burning types of pain with vertigo, worse in the morning. Stools are hard, dry, knotty. Rectum is sore, dry and inflamed with paretic condition. Women of sedentary habits are constipated and they have leucorrhoea. Alumina is suited to constitutionally chilly patients.

Low spirited patients are afraid they will lose reason. Time passes too slowly. Suicidal tendency when she sees knife or blade.

MODALITIES :

- < In general in the morning, by cold.
- > Open air, by washing the parts with cold water, warm room.

1.1.2 BORAX

Leucorrhoea is like white of an egg. With sensation as if hot fluid is flowing through genitalia. Menses are too soon, profuse, with griping pain in abdomen. These pains extend to small of back. Leucorrhoea especially after menses. Membranous dysmenorrhoea with pain in the breast during menses indicate this remedy. The psychological factor plays an important role other than the general causes of ill health and under-nutrition.There are other causes also.The patient is extremely anxious. Anxious about the future. Severe stitching pains in epigastric region with aphthae. White fungus-like growth in the mouth. Psoriatic condition of the skin with erysipelas on face. Herpes. Voluptuous dreams, cannot sleep on account of heat. Feeling of cobwebs on hands with itching of back of fingers, joints and hands.

Patient is very anxious especially from motions which have a downward direction. Anxious expressions on the face during the downward motion. When lies down, throws the hands up as if afraid of falling. Excessively nervous, easily frightened, very sensitive to sudden noises.

MODALITIES :

- < From downward motion, noise, warm weather, after menses.
- > Washing the parts with cold water, in the evening, by pressure.

1.1.3 KREOSOTUM

Corrosive itching within the vulva during the flow of leucorrhoea. Burning and swelling of labia with violent itching between labia and thighs. Before puberty poor general health, unclean personal hygiene with anaemia cause leucorrhoea. Discharges are yellow, acrid and with odour of green corn. Worse between menses. The menses are too early, prolonged and intermittent. Leucorrhoea is offensive and also intermittent.

Hoarseness of voice with pain in larynx which is worse in evening. Winter cough of old females with pressure on sternum. Dragging backache extending to genitalia and down to thighs. Abdomen is distended. Burning haemorrhoids. Urine is offensive. Violent itching of vulva and vagina. Worse after urination. Dreams of urinating. Enuresis in the first part of night. Patient has to hurry when there is desire for urination.

Mentally the patient is timid and anxious. Music causes palpitation. Sudden blackout of thoughts. Stupid, forgetful, peevish and irritable. Patient wants many things but throws away when given.

MODALITIES :

< Cold food, cold drinks, cold in general, cold applications, rest, open air, while lying, after menstrual flow.

> Warmth in general, hot drinks, hot food, by movements.

1.1.4 NATRUM MURIATICUM

Prolapse of the uterus causes cervical erosion, and chronic cervicitis. These are the two common causes of leucorrhoea. Parous women, during the child bearing period, become the victim of this disease. There is acute trichomonas and monilial vaginitis or chronic vaginitis especially in presence of a pessary and genital prolapse. Pelvic inflammatory diseases also play an important role. Use of the oral contraceptives may cause leucorrhoea. Menses are irregular, which are usually profuse in nature. Leucorrhoea is acrid, watery, worse in the morning. Cutting type of pain in urethra. Ineffectual labour-like pain with the suppressed menses. Leucorrhoea is white in the beginning but turns green afterwards. The patient is very sensitive as far as genitalia is concerned due to dryness of vagina.

Periodicity is well marked in this remedy and the symptoms are worse usually from 10 to 11 a.m. Marasmus or emaciation even though patient lives well. It is due to faulty assimilation. Patient craves for salt. She is thirsty, and has unquenchable thirst for cold water and feels better after drinking the same.

Mentally the patient is sad and melancholic due to suppression of grief, anger and desires. Disappointed love. Irresistible laughs for long time or at unsuitable time, followed by weeping mood. Consolation aggravates the sufferings. Forgetfulness, weak mind, forgets what she was about to say.

MODALITIES :

< Heat of sun, 10 - 11 a.m., at seashore, after mental exertion.

> Open air, lying down.

1.1.5 PLATINA

Bearing down sensation with prolapse of uterus. Inflammatory conditions of ovaries and fallopian tubes. Genitalia are oversensitive. In post-menopausal women, uterine polyps, decubitus ulcer and prolapse of uterus are responsible for leucorrhoea. Uterine fibroids and uterine carcinoma are also important factors for leucorrhoea. Leucorrhoea during parturition causes violent cramps in limbs and profuse haemorrhage, with hysterical and puerperal convulsion.

It is predominantly a women's remedy, especially suited to a hysterial woman, with uterine troubles. The ailments are due to shock, excitement, disappointment, grief, fright etc. Violent cramp-like pains which increase gradually and subside gradually. Bowels are constipated with colicky pain in abdomen.

Mental symptoms always alternate with physical symptoms. Patient generally is a hysterical woman. Thinks that she is superior and all others are inferior to her. Alternating moods. At one moment she laughs and next moment she is sad and weepy. Becomes serious and irritable at silly matters. Religious insanity.

MODALITIES :

< On standing and sitting.

> Walking in open air.

1.1.6 SILICEA

Leucorrhoea instead of menses. Milky, acrid leucorrhoea during urination. There is intense itching of vulva and vagina. The parts are very sensitive. Discharge of blood between menstrual periods. Discharge of bloody secretions every time when the child is nursed. Vaginal cyst is probably the cause of leucorrhoea. Deficiency of animal heat. The patient is usually oversensitive and weak. There is lack of assimilation, therefore patient suffers from anaemia. Catarrhal condition of the uterus and genital tract due to puerperal cervical erosion and granulation. Cervical, perineal tear is the cause of leucorrhoea.

Catarrhal condition of the respiratory tract. Hoarseness with dry and teasing cough. Tendency to take cold very easily. Desires cold drink and cold food. Dyspepsia with weak stomach. Waterbrash and vomiting more in the morning. Paralytic weakness of the extremities. Feet are icy cold. Corns on the soles. Constipation due to inability of rectum to evacuate and paralytic weakness of rectum.

The patient is nervous, excitable and sensitive to all impressions. There is lack of confidence and stamina. There is dread of appearing in public, especially in public speakers, want of grit.

MODALITIES :

< Full moon, new moon, uncovering, cold in general, lying on damp place, during menses.

> Warmth in general, summer, wrapping up of head.

1.1.7 HELONIAS

Leucorrhoea with severe burning and itching in the vulval region. Feeling of weight and soreness in the womb. Pruritus vulva. Severe backache after the discharges. Dragging pains in sacral region with prolapse. Leucorrhoea is thick and yellow, especially after miscarriage. Genital parts are hot, red and swollen. Sensation of weakness, dragging and weight in the sacrum and pelvis with great prostration are keynote indications for this remedy. There is tendency to prolapse and other malformations of uterus. Menses are often suppressed.

Albuminuria during pregnancy and at the time of menopause. Sensation as if a cold wind streamed up to calf of legs. Feet feel numb when sitting.

MODALITIES :

< Thinking of the complaints, motion, touch.

> Keeping herself busy.

Other important remedies for Leucorrhoea are

1. CANTHARIS
2. ACONITE
3. THUJA
4. CAUSTICUM
5. LACHESIS

==============

TOPIC 2

DYSMENORRHOEA

1.2.1 CIMICIFUGA

This remedy predominantly suits spasmodic dysmenorrhoea. Patient complaints of pain in lower abdomen which usually starts on first day of menstruation. Pains persist until the flow ceases. The victims are usually young unmarried females. Many times the uterus is not developed properly. Bearing down sensation with pressing pains in uterine region. Pains are shifting from one hip to another. Menses are suppressed or scanty and are offensive, with backache. Nervousness during menstruation. Menstrual blood is blackish and partly clotted. The flow does not ameliorate the pain.

The muscular pains are associated with uterine disturbances. It especially acts upon the patient of dysmenorrhoea with rheumatic complaints. Soreness and stiffness of back and neck. Restless feeling in limbs. Ovarian neuralgia. Shooting and throbbing pain in the head followed by nausea and vomiting.

Mentally the patient is greatly depressed. Mental symptoms are worse during menses and usually are alternating with rheumatic pains. Patient is always sad and hysterical. Wild feeling in brain. Headache after mental exertion and uterine discharge. All the mental as well as physical symptoms aggravated by menstrual flow is the important characteristic of Cimicifuga.

MODALITIES :

< In the morning, cold atmosphere, during menses and as the menstrual flow increases.

> By warmth in general, rest.

1.2.2 CAULOPHYLLUM

This is again a suitable remedy for spasmodic dysmenorrhoea. The patient has lack of tonicity of the womb. Before and during menstruation, there are spasmodic pains and patient complains that they fly in all directions. Great atony of the muscles of uterus, therefore the discharges stagnate in uterine cavity. Uterus is ill developed or it is smaller than the normal uterus. Cervical os is rigid and cervical meatus is pinhole. Pains are intermittent and come in paroxysms. With spasmodic pains of dysmenorrhoea the patient also complains of spasms of stomach with dyspepsia. There is stiffness of small joints of fingers, toes, ankles etc. Cutting and throbbing pains on flexing the fingers. These pains make the patient to change her position every few minutes.

Mentally the patient is fearful and hysterical. She is restless. Easily excitable.

MODALITIES :

< Cold, open air.

> Rest, warmth.

1.2.3 XANTHOXYLUM

The action of this remedy is usually on the mucous membrane of uterus and it also acts on ovary. The menses are too early and too painful. Usually associated with ovarian neuralgia with pain in loins and lower abdomen. The pains are agonising and shooting which start in left loin and travel down the thighs. Neuralgic dysmenorrhoea is well treated by this remedy. Menses are thick, almost black. Leucorrhoea at the time of menses.

Neurasthenic patients who are thin, emaciated with poor assimilation and insomnia, with occipital headache are well treated by this remedy.

With dysmenorrhoea there are griping pains in abdomen with diarrhoea. Patient has aphonia and has desire to take long breath. Weakness or paralysis, especially of left side, followed by spinal disorders. Patient has rheumatic affections.

Neuralgic, shooting pains as if from electric current. Sleep is disturbed due to pains.

Mentally the patient is nervous, depressed and frightened. Does not wish to express herself.

MODALITIES :

< In all the positions; warmth in general, mental exertion.

> In open air.

1.2.4 VIBURNUM OPULUS

This is a useful remedy in spasmodic and membranous dysmenorrhoea when the menses are too late, scanty and lasting for few hours. Menses are offensive and are associated with severe cramps in legs. Bearing down pains in the uterine region. Tearing and shooting pain in ovarian region. On examination, the parts are found congested and oedematous. Excoriating leucorrhoea which causes itching of genitalia. Patient complains of pain in back, radiating to loins and womb which are more in the early morning.

Uterine complaints associated with cramps in thighs, extending to calf, is the keynote of this remedy. Colicky pain in the pelvic region. Lower extremities are stiff and sore with sensation of weakness and heaviness. Patient has frequent urging for urination.

Mentally the patient is irritable with vertigo. She feels as if falling forward.

MODALITIES :

< On lying, in a warm room, morning.

> Open air, evening.

1.2.5 MELILOTUS ALBA

This is an indicated remedy for congestive and spasmodic dysmenorrhoea. Congestion is seen along the genital tract. Congestion of the uterine mucous membrane, of the ovaries, of the fallopian tubes, which makes the patient restless. This congestion may produce neuritic pains and paraethesia. Menses are scanty and intermittent. Flow starts, stops and reappears after a gap of ten to fifteen days or so. Striking pains in external genitalia. Ovarian neuralgia.

Throbbing headache with nausea and vomiting. Sense of pressure over the orbits. Hands and feet are cold. Black spots before the eyes. Eyes are heavy; blurred sight; wants to close the eyes tightly to get relief. Pain in knee joints, patient wants to stretch the legs. But this does not relieve the pain. Numbness of lower extremities with pain in knee joints.

Mentally she is forgetful and unable to fix the mind. Wants to run away and to hide. Delusions. Thinks everyone is looking at her. Patient has fear to talk in loud voice.

MODALITIES :

< In rainy season, change of weather, by motion.

> By cold, rest, pressure.

1.2.6 COLOCYNTH

Colocynth is an indicated remedy where patient complains of severe neuralgic pains along the course of nerves. The nerve plexus of the ovary or uterus is affected which gives agonising pains with great restlessness. Left sided ovary is usually affected. Burning pains in the ovary. The pains are better by hard pressure and heat. The affected parts become numb with pricking and tingling sensations. Pains are more after eating and after anger. Dysmenorrhoea with copious bleeding.

The patient is thirsty. Appetite is reduced, sometimes there is aversion to food. Colicky pain in abdomen after eating which, sometimes results in nausea and vomiting. Patient retches after vomiting till pain subsides. There is also neuralgic pain in head. Violent periodical or intermittent headache. Left sided sciatica may be the associated symptom.

MODALITIES :

< Evening, after anger, cold, after eating.

> Hot fermentation, hard pressure, bending double.

1.2.7 BELLADONNA

Congestive dysmenorrhoea is well marked in this remedy. Congestion of the endometrium, ovaries, fallopian tubes, cervix, etc. Thus in short there is severe inflammation and the parts become very sensitive. Vagina is dry and hot. Dragging pains around the loins. Severe throbbing in sacrum. Profuse menstrual bleeding which is bright red in colour. Haemorrhages are hot. Uterus is sore and irritated.

This is an acute and short acting remedy. Sudden and violent onset is the keynote of this remedy. Pains come suddenly and disappear suddenly. Inflammatory conditions of the body or particular organ with violent pains and intense heat mark this remedy. The affected parts are red and sore. Throbbing of the affected part is another characteristic of this remedy. Head is red, hot, burning and congested with rush of blood to head. Dryness of mouth. Tongue is dry and bright red.

Mental symptoms are usually associated with high fever. Hallucinations, delirium, frightful images. The patient becomes wild and violent. She strikes, bites and tears the clothes. When the pains subside, patient goes into semicomatose state. All the mental symptoms are usually associated with heat, burning and restlessness.

MODALITIES :

< Touch, motion, cold air.

> Rest, warm room.

Other useful remedies for dysmenorrhoea are

1) CHAMOMILLA
2) APIS. MEL
3) LAPIS ALBUS
4) NATRUM MUR
5) BORAX
6) USTILAGO
7) LYCOPODIUM

==============

TOPIC 3

MENORRHAGIA

1.3.1 IODUM

Menorrhagia due to endocrinal dysfunction is well treated by this remedy, especially of the thyroid gland. The synthesis of thyroxine is hampered in these patients. Menstruation is irregular. Generally it is uterine haemorrhage. Menorrhagia with enlarged and indurated uterus. Iodum may be thought of when haemorrhage is due to pathological condition of uterus. There is acute catarrh of endometrium. Great weakness during menses, wedge-like pain in right ovarian region. Haemorrhage occurring at every stool with cutting pain in the abdomen, pain in the loins and small of back.

Patient shows signs of rapid metabolism. Loss of flesh with great appetite. Majority of glands of the body are hypertrophied, hard and nodular. Patient is emaciated. Hot patient, better by cold. Patient wants to move all the time as the symptoms are relieved when she is busy. Patient is always hungry and wants to eat all the time. But also has indigestion with diarrhoea. Assimilation is poor and is very low. Liver and spleen are enlarged. Incontinence of urine. Cough with difficulty in breathing. Catarrhal condition of the nose. Watery discharges with sneezing.

Patient is weak minded and forgetful. Impulsive insanity. Sadness with melancholic mood. Excitable restlessness and very anxious. Patient has the impulse of doing something in a hurry.

MODALITIES :

< Warmth in general, exertion.

> Eating, cold in general, by walking or by movement.

1.3.2 PHOSPHORUS

Pelvic inflammatory diseases such as chronic salpingo-oophoritis, chronic endometritis usually tubercular in origin or malignancy of genito-urinary tract is well treated by this remedy. Dysfunctional uterine haemorrhage is an important cause of menorrhagia. Polycystic ovarian disease may be seen developed if the patient has sycosis as a predominant miasm. Menses too early and scanty but last too long. Stitching pains. Bleeding is copious, dark red and non-coagulable. Menorrhagia in nursing women, burning and stitching pain in the region of uterus. Ovaries are inflamed and painful at the time of menses. These pains are radiating down the inner side of the thighs. Fibroids of the uterus are common. Menorrhagia due to uterine polypi.

There is numbness, trembling and paralytic weakness of the extremities. Major joints of the body are inflamed and stiff. Stitching pains in the breast during menses. Laryngitis with hoarseness of voice. Bronchitis with bloody expectoration. Sharp and stitching pain in chest with haemoptysis. Left side of the chest is usually affected. Haemorrhoids with burning pain. Morning diarrhoea, stools are profuse, watery and involuntarily poured with a sensation as if anus is wide open.

Mentally patient is excitable and has violent imaginations which prevent the sleep. Patient is hypersensitive to external impressions. Great debility and prostration, weak memory. Anxiety, irritability and fear mark the remedy. Stupor, dizziness, sluggishness and delirious condition of the patient. Brain fag from mental exertion.

MODALITIES :

< Evening, on the left side, cold in general.

> Warmth in general, lying on right side.

1.3.3 SABINA

It is great anti-haemorrhagic remedy. Sabina acts upon the mucous membrane of the uterus and also upon the serous and fibrous membranes. Pains fly from sacrum to pubis. Haemorrhage is profuse at the time of menses. They are long lasting, partly fluid and partly clotted, offensive in nature. Blood comes in gushes. Intense colicky pains in abdomen at the time of menses, these pains are associated with bearing down or labour-like pains. Pains traverse from vagina to uterus. Discharges of blood between periods with sexual excitement. Inflammation of the tubes, ovaries and uterus. Uterine fibroids are usually the cause of menorrhagia at the climacteric age. Profuse leucorrhoea and the discharge is bloody.

Sabina patient has haemorrhagic tendency and bleeds from all the mucous membranes. Pulsation all over the body with sense of fulness. Shooting type of pains from sacrum to pubes. Sense of fulness in the rectum with bleeding haemorrhoids and the blood is bright red. Warts around the anus, pus-like gonorrhoeal discharge from urethra. Urethra is inflamed.

Patient is nervous, sad and depressed. Music makes her nervous. Also music is intolerable for her.

MODALITIES :

< Warmth in general, warm room, hot food, warm applications.

> Cold open air, cold drinks, cold applications.

1.3.4 CIMICIFUGA

Menorrhagia due to prolapse of uterus. Menses are profuse and too early, sometimes twice a month. Blood is dark, coagulated. There is bearing down and pressing pains in the uterine region. This pain traverse from hip to hip. Severe pains in lower extremities. Backache after menstruation, with heavy, pressing down sensation. If the menses are suppressed, they are scanty or copious with severe pains during the flow. All the symptoms either physical or mental are worse during menses. Discharges are offensive. Spasms and cramps in the muscles of back. Shooting and throbbing pains in head as a reflex of uterine bleeding. Nausea and vomiting caused by pressure on the spine. Ovarian neuralgia is well treated by this remedy. Pains across the pelvis. Rheumatic pains in joints. Sleeplessness.

Patient is depressed. Visions of rat, mice running across the room. Delirium, hysterical and epileptic spasms. The mental symptoms are intermingled with rheumatism. Mental symptoms are worse during menses. Sabina patient is so much depressed that, she cries when questioned. Sensation as if some weight is laid on her head. Almost all the symptoms are due to fear and she is worse during menstrual flow.

MODALITIES :

< During menses; in cold season; cold drinks.

> Warmth in general, after menstrual flow.

1.3.5 KREOSOTE

Endometrial polyps or the abnormal growths of the uterine cavity is the fundamental cause of menorrhagia. Burning and soreness in external and internal parts. Menses are too early, prolonged and the flow is black and offensive. The discharges excoriate the thighs. Leucorrhoea before menses, which is yellow, acrid, excoriating and offensive. Bleeding from uterine cavity is continuous in nature, and the flow increases on exertion.

Patient complains of pain in abdomen, especially before the menstruation. Burning and scratching sensation at vulval region and medial sides of thighs. Sudden desire for urination. Patient is not in a position to hold the urine and she has to hurry for urination. Fulness and burning pain in the stomach. Nausea ends in vomiting. This drug can be used for the palliation of malignancy of genital organs. All symptoms worse at the time of menses is the key-note symptom of this drug. All the mucous membranes of the body are raw and inflamed with bleeding and ulceration. All the discharges of the body are very offensive.

Patient is very irritable during menses. Patient desires many things, but is not satisfied with those when she gets them. Always unsatisfied. Music makes her weep.

MODALITIES :

< Cold in general; cold air; after washing the parts.

> Warmth in general, rest in bed.

1.3.6 BELLADONNA

Menses in case of Belladonna are increased and premature. Along with the menorrhagia, she complains of mastodynia. The menses are profuse and bright red in colour due to excess of blood. There are cutting pains from hip to hip. Blood is very dark and offensive and feels hot, with dark clots. Strong bearing down pain she feels as if everything would escape from the vagina.

Belladonna patient is very chilly and easily affected by draught of air. She has violent congestion in her body so she feels very hot in every parts. Redness, heat and burning are the red strands for this remedy. She becomes hyper-sensitive during ailments. She is drowsy or sleepy but cannot sleep due to the intolerable pains associated with each symptom. There is great dryness everywhere, still she does not like to drink water.

Mentally she has marked violence due to turmoil in her brain from congestion. She tears the clothes, bites and strikes everybody. Delirium, unconciousness. Illusion, delusion and hallucination. Her face is shiny red and very hot; pupils are dilated. Throbbing of each and every vessel during the flow.

MODALITIES :

< Draught of air, heat of sun, moving about, bending, lying down.

> Sitting in erect position.

1.3.7 PLATINA

Menses in case of Platina lady are much earlier, too profuse but their duration may be short or long. The blood is very dark and clotted. Spasmodic pains. Pains come and go gradually. Severe bearing down with numbness of pelvic organs. She feels very chilly. Flow may appear every fourteenth day. She has tingling sensation in the parts. After menses there is profuse leucorrhoea.

Platina is known for hyperaesthesia leading to vaginismus and nymphomania. The parts are sensitive to touch and go into spasm on touch. Colicky pains in abdomen. Paralytic weakness with chilliness and numbness in the parts. Headache with sense of constriction in the scalp. Constipated even with soft stool. She is very hot patient. She cannot complete the coition due to vaginismus.

Mentally she has her own peculiar symptoms. She is hysterical, sanguine and proud. Superiority complex, treats others as minor personalities. She has increased sexual appetite. Anxiety, talks very little and has great fear of death.

MODALLITIES :

< By rest, on excitement, while sitting and standing.

> Moving in open air.

Other important remedies for menorrhoea are

1. RHUS TOXICODENDRON
2. SECALE CORNUTUM
3. CINNAMONUM
4. ARSENICUM ALBUM
5. NUX VOMICA

===============

TOPIC 4

METRORRHAGIA

1.4.1 PLUMBUM METALLICUM

Patients are of climacteric age group. Bleeding probably might be due to fibroids of the uterus or due to other systemic diseases such as hypertension, supressed eruptions and progressive muscular atrophy. Bleeding is in the form of dark clots which sometimes alternates with frank blood and serum. There is great vaginismus. Vulva and vagina are hypersensitive. Metrorrhagia also may be due to incomplete abortion and patient complains of intermittent bleeding for days together. There is sensation of a string pulling from abdomen to back. Dark clots difficult to expel from cervical os, thus there is severe pain in abdomen.

This drug is useful in general sclerotic conditions. Hypertension due to atherosclerosis is marked. Constrictive and boring pains. Excessive colicky pains radiating to uterine region.

Patient is confused and has great mental depression, unable to remember the incidences. Patient thinks that her confused state will be observed by other persons; thus she is very timid. Broods on past events. Patient is in delirious condition.

MODALITIES :

< After movements, at night times.

> By hard pressure.

1.4.2 TRILLIUM

This is the remedy used for active uterine haemorrhage, especially after hormonal imbalance. Patients are of different age groups and the menstrual flow starts after about 7-10 days of previous menstrual cycle. Bleeding continues, in the intervals of 7-10 days followed by great prostration. This remedy acts well for women who unceasingly bleed after parturition or miscarriage. Sometimes bleeding starts at climacteric. Gushing of bright red blood from the uterus, later on the blood becomes pale due to anaemia. Menses often come from overexertion, too long ride etc. Profuse flow, attended with faint feeling in epigastric region. Extremities cold; rapid and feeble pulse.

This is predominantly a general haemorrhagic remedy. Patient complains of great faintness and dizziness. Chronic diarrhoea associated with bloody mucus is well treated by this remedy. Uterine haemorrhage may be due to threatened abortion. Relaxation of pelvic organs. Cramplike pains in calf muscles. Cough with spitting of blood. Expectoration is purulent and copious. Pains at the sternal end. Suffocative attack of irregular breathing with sneezing. Shooting pains in the chest.

Patient is nervous and melancholic. She has lost all hopes. She has a peculiar tendency of negative thinking.

MODALITIES :

< Movements, clothings, heat of sun, after covering.

> Rest, cold, open air.

1.4.3 SECALE COR

Profuse, painless bleeding in the women of the climacteric age group. Secale cor is hot patient and thus patients from tropical regions respond well to this remedy. Passive haemorrhage and blood is dark coloured, seldom clots. Discharges are offensive and scanty. Motion aggravates the flow. This remedy is suitable where the weakness is not caused by loss of blood. Haemorrhage with strong and spasmodic contraction of uterus. Every flow preceded by strong bearing down pains. Haemorrhage due to atony of uterus as in protracted labour or miscarriage. Menses are usually too profuse and long-lasting.

Severe anaemic condition of the patient. Coldness, numbness, petechiae, mortification with gangrene. Useful remedy for old women who are thin and scrawny. All the Secale cor conditions are better by cold. Continuous oozing of watery black blood from lesions. Excessive thirst. Pale, pinched, sunken face with livid spots on it. Coldness and cramps in lower extremities after cholera-like stools. Hands and feet are cold and dry.

Secale cor decreases the secretions and flow of pancreatic juice and thus there is hypertension. Patient is restless and irritable. Sluggish, slow in movements, cannot decide if the choice is given. Forgetful, confused.

MODALITIES :

- < Heat in general, warmth, covering the parts.
- > Cold application, cold in general, rubbing the extremities, pressure on abdomen.

1.4.4 ARSENICUM ALBUM

Profuse long-lasting blood flow from the uterus in women who are thin, feeble and cachectic. Pain or bleeding or any disorganization of uterus or ovaries with great debility, restlessness and lancinating, burning pains in uterus. The uterus is larger and softer than usual which dilates the blood vessels, causing excessive haemorrhage. Bleeding is excessive and too soon. Offensive leucorrhoea before bleeding sets in. Sensation as if pains in uterus arise from red hot wires. They are worse from least exertion. Bleeding causes great fatigue. Patient is better in warm room. Menorrhagia after abortion.

Patient is anxious and restless. Fear of death, afraid when left alone. Hallucinations of smell and sight. Patient is selfish and lacks courage. Patient is very much sensitive to slightest disorder and is confused. Fear of death, patient thinks that it is useless to take the medicines.

Patient cannot bear smell or sight of food. Great

unquenchable thirst for little quantity of cold water at shorter intervals. Nausea, retching. Vomiting after eating or drinking. Long-lasting eructations. Small, offensive dark stools with much prostration, worse at night and after eating and drinking. Headache is relieved by cold application, when other symptoms are aggravated by cold. Air passage is constricted. Thus patient has asthma which is worse at midnight. Sleep is disturbed. Could sleep a little when head is raised on pillow. High degree of fever, where periodicity is well marked.

MODALITIES :

- < In wet weather, after midnight, from cold applications, cold drinks.
- > Heat in general, warm drinks, rest.

1.4.5 THLASPI BURSA

This is an anti-haemorrhagic remedy. The patients are prone to develop fibroids or abnormal growth in the uterine cavity. Uterine bleeding with cramps in lower extremities. Bleeding is in the form of clots. This remedy acts well in condition where there is suppression of uterine disease. Metrorrhagia due to intramural fibroid of uterus is well treated by this remedy when used in low potency. As cervical os is small or closed there is great difficulty to expel the clots. This expulsion of clots can be done by this remedy. Pains and bleeding are excessive alternately. In attempt to expel the clots, the uterus contracts, thus pains are more. Too frequent periods, with profuse bleeding. Uterus is very sore, therefore causes severe pains. Bruised feeling in pelvic region.

Frank blood from all the orifices such as nose, mouth, ears etc. There is frequent desire for urination. Patient usually complains of dysuria. Haematuria due to any reason is well treated by this remedy.

1.4.6 PULSATILLA

Dark, coagulated blood emitted in paroxysms during the period of metrorrhagia. Before periods, there is leucorrhoea which is acrid, burning and creamy in nature. Backache associated with bleeding. Labour-like pains at the time of menses. Type of blood ever changing. The mucous membrane of uterus is affected. The genitalia are very sensitive. Tardy menses which are too late, scanty, thick, dark, clotted. Chilliness and nausea with bearing down pains at the time of menses. Crampy pains in abdomen. Diarrhoea during and after menses.

Suitable for thin, fair, beautiful ladies with sandy hair and blue eyes. Patient complains of greasy taste in mouth. Dry mouth without thirst. Crack in middle of lower lip. Foul smell from mouth. Eructations after fatty food. Dyspepsia with great tightness after meal. All-gone sensation in abdomen especially in tea-drinkers. Hoarseness of voice with dry cough in evening and at night. Must sit up in the bed to get relief. Urine emitted with cough. Drawing, tensive pains in thighs and legs with restlessness. Pain in legs with cramps in calf muscles. Urticaria after rich food, followed by diarrhoea.

Mentally the patient is mild, gentle and yielding disposition. Sad, cries while narrating the complaints. Changeability is well marked. Timid, fears in the evening and to be alone, likes sympathy.

MODALITIES :

< From heat in general, rich fatty food, after eating, towards evening, warmth.

> Open air, movements, cold drinks, cold food.

1.4.7 ALETRIS FARINOSA

This is the remedy suitable for women who bleed and bleed and become victims of anaemia. Metrorrhagia due to prolapse of the uterus as the pelvic organs are relaxed. Procedentia causes intermittent, profuse haemorrhage. Due to continuous bleeding, patient seems to be tired all the time. Due to prolapse, secondary infection sets in causing leucorrhoea, cervical ulcers etc. Metrorrhagia in chlorotic girls and pregnant women can be treated well by this remedy. Menses are premature and profuse with labour-like pains. Uterus seems to be heavy with pain in right inguinal region.

Patients are anaemic due to severe blood loss and thus prone to infectious diseases and leucorrhoea. The patient has tendency for habitual abortion.

Other important remedies for metrorrhagia are

1) CACTUS GRANDIFLORA
2) CALCAREA CARB
3) CINNAMONUM
4) NITRIC ACID
5) VINCA MINOR
6) AMBRA GRISEA

================

TOPIC 5

AMENORRHOEA

1.5.1 AGNUS CASTUS

Obesity with hypogonadism may manifest with primary amenorrhoea. Menses are suppressed with violent and contracting pains especially in lower abdomen. Low sexual vitality as patient is sexually melancholic. Relaxation of genitalia with leucorrhoea.

Patient complains of nausea with sensation as if intestines were pressed downwards, sinking down, with strong desire to support them.

Mentally patient is melancholic, as far as sex is concerned. Patient is sad and depressed. Intense fear of death. Constant thinking, thus absent-minded. Patient is forgetful and therefore lacks confidence. Lost interest in sex as she is always nervous and depressed.

MODALITIES :

< Cold, thinking of the problems, when alone.

> In warm weather, at rest, company.

1.5.2 LYCOPODIUM

Suppression of menses from fright, sadness, which develops anorexia nervosa. Amenorrhoea as a result of psychosomatic trauma. Manifested by morbidly being afraid of something. Marked anorexia. Loses weight, extreme emaciation results into amenorrhoea.

Amenorrhoea may be secondary to diseases of central

nervous system as meningitis, epilepsy etc. Patient has fainting fits with sour taste; sour eructations and sour vomiting. Menses are too late, last too long and too profuse. Vagina is dry which makes coition painful. Pain in the region of ovary, specially right sided. Leucorrhoea is acrid with burning in vagina.

Patient has dyspepsia due to fried and fermentable food. Patient desires sweet things. Food tastes sour, sour eructations. Throbbing headache with vertigo in morning, on rising. Patient presents with greyish yellow colour of face with blue circles around the eyes. Patient is emaciated in upper part and semidropsical in lower region.

Mentally patient is melancholic and afraid to be alone. Apprehensive, weak memory with confused thoughts, loss of self-confidence.

MODALITIES :

< Right side, from right to left, between 4 - 8 p.m.; from heat, in warm room, hot air, warm applications.

> By movements, after midnight, on getting cold, from being uncovered.

1.5.3 PULSATILLA

Amenorrhoea due to getting feet wet, nervous debility or chlorosis. Faulty gonadal development results into too late, scanty and thick, dark menses. Acrid leucorrhoea instead of menses which is burning and creamy. Menarchae delayed in chlorotic girls. Epistaxis instead of menses. Vicarious menstruation.

Patient has great aversion to fatty food, hot drinks and warm food. Eructations, taste of food remains in mouth for longer time. Changeability of symptoms. Dry mouth without thirst. Dry cough, copious mucous expectoration. Pain in limbs shifting rapidly.

Mentally patient has weeping disposition. Easily discouraged, very emotional, wants company, fears to be alone in evening, wants sympathy from others. Consolation ameliorates her complaints. Fear of meeting persons of opposite sex.

MODALITIES :

< Heat, rich fatty food, eating, evening, warm room, lying on left or painless side.

> Motion, open air, cold applications, cold food and cold drinks, consolation.

1.5.4 CIMICIFUGA [ACTAEA RACEMOSA]

Amenorrhoea due to ovarian disorders, such as polycystic ovarian disease; obesity and hirsutism. Amenorrhoea may also be due to congenital adrenal hyperplasia which shows precocious virilism. There is irritation in ovaries due to ovarian disorders. Pain in the ovarian region, shoots upwards and downwards, on anterior side of thighs. Ovarian neuralgia.

Patient complains of sinking in epigastrium with nausea and vomiting. Asthenopia associated with pelvic troubles. Shooting pain in eyes; photophobia. Spine is very sensitive, stiffness of back. Dry, short cough with scanty secretions.

Mentally she is disturbed with sensation as if cloud has enveloped her head. Great depression with dreams of impending evil. Visions of rats. Mania following disappearance of neuralgia. Hysterical woman in puerperal mania where there is physiological amenorrhoea.

MODALITIES :

< Morning, cold.

> Warmth, after eating.

1.5.5 SEPIA

Amenorrhoea due to relaxed pelvic organs. Bearing down sensation, as if everything would escape through vulva, thus must cross her legs to prevent protrusion or has to press against vulva. Leucorrhoea is yellow, greenish with much itching. Sharp clutching pains. Violent stitches upwards in the vagina, from uterus to umbilicus. Prolapse of uterus and vagina. Male type of pelvis, gonadal dysfunction. Karyotype, musculine look.

Patient looks pale, anaemic. Earthy complexion, yellowish discolouration. Brown patches on the cheeks. Cachectic, yellow face or "tell-tale face." Chronic catarrhal condition of nose. There is nausea and milky vomiting, worse in the morning. Has to strain great, for stools. Constant urging for urination. Urine is milky. Burning pain during urination.

Patient is hysterical and indifferent. Has no more affection for whom she loved best. Cannot narrate her complaints without weeping. Sad and gentle at a moment but becomes excitable and obstinate in next moment. Consolation aggravates her complaints.

MODALITIES :

< Getting feet wet, after washing, laundry work, damp wet weather, in the evening.

> Movements, hard pressure, warmth, after sleep.

1.5.6 SENECIO AUREUS

Patients are usually young girls, where functional amenorrhoea is observed. Causative factors are malnutrition and hormonal imbalance. Thus in such cases the basic fundamental cause is to be removed or to be treated so as to start menses. These particular patients have anaemia with malabsorption syndrome. This remedy acts well where inflammation of genital organs is seen with amenorrhoea. Menses are suppressed or retarded.

Acute inflammatory conditions of upper respiratory tract. Hoarseness of voice with inflammatory condition of genito-urinary tract. Patient usually complains of scanty and high coloured urine.

Mentally patient is timid, worried, nervous, despondent and cannot fix her mind on one subject. Restless so cannot complete any task.

MODALITIES :

< Before menses, while ascending.

> Start of flow, after stools.

1.5.7 NATRUM MURIATICUM

Menses are suppressed usually due to prolonged consumption of excessive salt. It causes profound nutritive changes in the system; like changes in the form of anasarca and also changes in the blood, causing anaemia and leucocytosis. These patients are greatly debilitated and feel profound weakness especially in morning. Menses are suppressed due to severe anaemia and debility. There is prolapse of urogenital system and dysfunction of the uterus takes place. There are cutting pains in the vaginal fornices. Leucorrhoea with chronic cervicitis. Bearing down pains, worse in the morning.

Patient may have complaints of pain in back with desire for firm support. Palms are hot and perspiring. Numbness and tingling in fingers. Frothy white coating on tongue, sense of dryness. Mapped tongue. Patient is hungry, eats well yet loses flesh. Cutting pain in abdomen. Dry eruptions on the skin. Greasy skin.

Mentally patient is frightful and angry. Amenorrhoea is due to ill effects of grieves. Patient is depressed. Consolation aggravates the condition. Patient wants to be alone and has great desire to cry.

MODALITIES :

< Noise, music, in warm room, at 10 a.m., mental exertion, heat.

> Open air, cold bathing, pressure against back or support to the back.

Other useful remedies for amenorrhoea are -

1. CUPRUM METALLICUM
2. CYCLAMEN
3. LOBELIA INFLATA
4. PHOSPHORUS
5. USTILAGO

****

CHAPTER - 2

DISEASES OF VULVA

TOPIC - 1

ACUTE VULVITIS

2.1.1 DULCAMARA

Herpetic eruptions can be well treated by this remedy. Dulcamara lady has psoric and sycotic trend. Thus she is prone to various skin eruptions, outgrowths and catarrhal inflammation of mucous membranes. This inflammation produces profuse secretion which causes intense irritation to the skin. Lady complains of vesicular eruptions at and around the vulval region, with desire to scratch until it bleeds.

Along with vulvitis there is urticarial rash all over the body without fever. Rash is on the back, abdomen and on hands. Patient has desire to scratch but this scratching is followed by intense burning. Catarrhal condition of nose, eyes and mucous membrane of gastrointestinal tract due to getting chilled in hot weather. Also there is catarrhal condition of bladder with urinary tract infections which results in vulvitis. Patient is prone to take cold and every cold settles in the mucous membrane causing inflammation. She has suppression of menses from working in damp, wet places. Appearance of rash can be seen before she menstruates. Dysmenorrhoea with blotches all over the body. Humid eruptions especially on cheeks and face. She has cough with free expectoration, tickling in larynx; whooping cough. Warts on the hands with perspiration on palms.

Patient is confused. All the complaints of Dulcamara lady are due to her working in damp, marshy places or basements

MODALITIES

< Cold in general, damp wet weather, cold drinks, cold food, cold air, when the days are hot and nights are cold. suppression of the sweat, getting wet.

> Moving about, parts washed with warm water, warm dry weather.

2.1.2 APIS MELLIFICA –

She has waxy skin which looks pale and oedematous. Cellular tissues of vulva are affected causing vulvitis. There are stinging pains, soreness and inflammation with redness of vulval region. With vulvitis, lady also complains of inflammation of the endometrium of uterus, oophoritis, right ovary is especially affected. Affections of Douglas's pouch; right side is very much sensitive. Vulval region has burning, stinging, tearing and cutting pains. Menses are suppressed usually in young girls. Burning and soreness while urinating. After inflammation of vulva there is chill with fever.

Apis lady always complains of migraine. Great redness of face. She has baglike swelling under lower eyelids. The eyelids are congested, swollen and oedematous with intense burning and stinging pains. Hot lachrymation with photophobia. Sore feeling in the stomach. Patient is thirstless. Craves milk. Fiery red tongue. Oedema of labia relieved by cold water. Metrorrhagia with profuse bleeding, with sense of heaviness in abdomen. Stinging pains in abdomen and viscera. She has hoarseness of voice, dyspnoea, breathing hurried and difficult. Erysipelas with sensitiveness and swelling. Patient is drowsy but fails to get sound sleep.

Lady is indifferent. Very awkward and drops the things readily from hands. Stupor with sudden sharp cries. She has erotic mania. She feels as if she will die. Wants to cry. Jealous.

Cannot concentrate the mind when attempts to read and study. Dreams are full of fear and toil. Dreams of flying. Unconciousness.

MODALITIES :

< Heat in general, during sleep, touch and wrapping, vexation.

> Cold in general, open air.

2.1.3 CALCAREA CARBONICA

Patient is having sycotic trend, therefore prone to get overgrowths and also she has tubercular diathesis, therefore postinfectious vulvitis is well treated by this remedy. Inflammation of the vulval region produces leucorrhoea which is milky white and acrid. It causes burning and itching of the parts. The parts are sore and least excitement causes return of leucorrhoea. Cutting pains in the uterus. Vulvitis in young girls and children is well treated by this remedy. Calcarea lady has early menarche, therefore cannot keep the parts clean, this results in trichomonal, monilial infections.

Patient is very chilly and takes cold easily. Every cold settles in throat. Tonsillitis with thick yellow mucus in throat. Crops of various skin eruptions. Dry, cracked skin with very much burning and itching. Gouty and rheumatic diathesis. Sore taste in the mouth, great thirst. Potbelly appearance of abdomen, looks like inverted saucer; very painful on pressure. Great craving for indigestible things. She has craving for eggs. She complains of habitual constipation. Patient feels much better when constipated. Dyspnoea with stitching pains in chest. Bones are soft and weak. As the constitution of patient is fat, fair and flabby, these bones cannot bear the weight of the body and therefore the curvatures of the bones.

Patient is sad and apprehensive. Fear of darkness. Anxiety with palpitation and restlessness of mind. Mental excitement causes profuse return of flow. Forgetful, gloomy and low spirited. Aversion to work.

MODALITIES

< Cold in any form, physical or mental work, standing, bathing, wet weather, full moon.

> Dry climate, lying on affected side.

2.1.4 XEROPHYLLUM

The lady is prone to soft tissue infection, these include furunculosis as a result of infection of hair follicle. There is infected sebaceous cyst, which results in vulvitis. Infected perineal wounds following operation or childbirth. Bartholinitis, skenitis and diphtheritic vulvitis can be best treated by this remedy. There is bearing down sensation with prolapse is of uterus. This prolapse many a time responsible for chronic irritation of vulva, which causes furious itching of vulval region. There is thick, yellowish, mucus-like discharge from infected part of vulva. The skin around vulva is cracked; feels like leather.

The lady is constipated and passes small amounts of stools at a time in the form of lumps. Stools are hard so she has to strain at stool. Tendency to pass flatus. She has increased sexual desire with pain in ovarian region and uterus.

Patient is dull and due to intense, furious itching fails to concentrate on a particular work. The mind is diverted and cannot remember the things properly. Fails to remember the names of the objects and friends. Fails to remember the spellings of common words. Writes last letter of the word first.

MODALITIES :

< Washing the part by cold water, in the afternoon, in the evening.

> Washing the part by hot water, in morning, moving around.

2.1.5 BELLADONNA

This patient has got active congestion of the vulval region. Acute inflammation of vulval region. Many a time there is pyogenic vulvitis. Parasitic infection like trichomona and bacterial vulvitis is best treated by this remedy. Acute and sudden attack is characteristic in Belladonna. Violence is well marked. Vulval region is red, hot and there is throbbing type of pain. The parts are very sensitive and there is sense of protrusion. Sensation as if the parts would prolapse from the region. Urethral orifice is sore, irritable and congested. Painful and very sensitive to touch. Sore, bruised feeling in the genitalia. Haematuria due to congestion. Uterus is congested and becomes very heavy due to which the uterine supports become weak. Thus prolapse of uterus with bearing down pains.

With vulvitis, there is inflammation of trachea, larynx. Throat is raw, sore and constricted. Cough without expectoration. Aphonia. Acute inflammation of gastro-intestinal tract with colicky pain in stomach, pains are ameliorated by bending double. Patient has constant urge for urination, dribbling of urine causes vulvitis. Sudden violent attack of fever with vulvitis. Congestion of head during fever. Skin is smooth and shiny, hot, burning; skin around the vulval region is very sensitive to touch.

Patient is wild and violent. Hallucinations and delusions, sees various things. Fear of imaginary things. Wants to keep herself away from those things. Horrible and fearful dreams. She gets frightened and wakes up from sleep.

MODALITIES :

< By movement, slightest touch, in the night times, hot season.

>Rest, in warm room.

2.1.6 MAGNESIA PHOSPHORICA

Vulvitis due to recurrent infections. Soreness and stiffness of parts. Patient often suffers from membranous dysmenorrhoea. Thus there is increased blood flow to external genitalia, i.e. vulval region and labia. Swelling of external parts with great sensitiveness. Ovaries are swollen, indurated and there is ovarian neuralgia. Vaginismus is also well treated by this remedy.

Spasms of stomach. Flatulent colic which makes the patient to bend double. Belching of gas with no reason. Fullness and bloated sensation in abdomen. She has to loosen clothing to get relief from abdominal discomfort. Colicky pain during menses. The pains in the vulval region are shooting, tearing and cutting. Thirst for very cold drinks. Involuntary shaking of hands.

Patient is lame all the time, especially during the attack. She is unable to think as she has mental diversions towards inflamed vulval region. Cannot concentrate her mind as the parts are very sore and sensitive.

MODALITIES :

< Washing the part with cold water, cold application.

> Heat, warmth, by hard pressure.

2.1.7 HEPAR SULPH

Hepar sulph. lady has tendency to suppuration. The inflamed parts are very sensitive to touch. This remedy has the power to localise the infection and to form the pus. The cellular tissues get infected due to chronic infections like gonorrhoea and other sexually transmitted diseases. Suppurative abscesses around the vulval region are very sensitive. Papules on the vulva, prone to suppuration. These ulcers bleed easily. Angioneuritic oedema is present on vulva with bloody suppuration, smells like old cheese. Patient sweats day and night without any relief from sufferings. Stitching and pricking sensation in the genitalia. Putrid ulcers surrounded by multiple papules.

Hepar sulph. lady is too much sensitive, with splinter-like pains in the genitalia. She craves sour things. Soreness, with ulcers in the genital area. Yellowish complexion. Middle of lower lip is cracked. Neuralgia of the right side, extending up to temporal region. Stitching pain in liver region. Aphonia. She craves acid things and strong tasting food, at the same time aversion to fatty food. Heaviness and distension with pressure on the stomach. Chronic and recurring urticaria.

Patient is anxious and very sensitive especially in evening and at night. She has thoughts of suicide. Trifle things irritate her mind. Sad and hopeless. Wants to speak hastily as she thinks that she will lose the words or break the link. Ferocious. Dejected. Anguish in evening.

MODALITIES :

< By cold, cold food, cold air, by touch, dry weather.

> Warmth in general, damp weather, from wrapping, after eating.

Other important remedies for acute vulvitis are

1. CANTHARIS
2. GRAPHITES
3. ACONITE
4. SULPHUR
5. LYCOPODIUM

==============

TOPIC 2

PRURITUS VULVA

2.2.1 CALADIUM SEGUINUM

Pruritus vulva especially during pregnancy and after miscarriage. There is inflammation of the vagina and the parts are very sore. Mucous discharge. Sebaceous cysts around the parts. Violent itching during mucous discharges, but as the parts are very sore, cannot scratch. There is no swelling but the parts are hot and sensitive. The parts are dry, scaly with violent corrosive itching. Crawling sensation in vagina. Voluptuous itching. Cramps in the uterus especially at night. There is violent itching in the external genitals which diverts her mental attention.

Coldness of single parts with nausea in the morning. Spasmodic cutting pains in the abdomen with intense tenderness on touch. Tongue is white coated. Sharp stitching in the right side of the chest. Oppression of breathing. Patient is drowsy and sleepy. She has rough and dry skin. Severe backache. She can hardly turn on the bed. Trembling of the limbs with pain in the calf muscles with pruritus.

Patient is forgetful and very much depressed. Due to pruritus vulva she is in an awkward position as neither she can sit comfortably and concentrate nor she can scratch as the parts are very sensitive and tender to touch. She is depressed and confused.

MODALITIES :

< Movement, closed rooms, after sweating, from 3 - 4 p.m. till midnight.

> In open air, movements and after a nap in afternoon.

2.2.2 PICRIC ACID

Picric acid lady complains of the inflammation of uterus, urethra and sometimes nephritis. This urinary tract infection passes to genitalia causing pruritus. Many a time lady is a known diabetic, urine contains sugar and albumin. Urine is loaded with uric acid, phosphates and urates. Enuresis is marked with dribbling of urine. This contaminated urine causes pruritus vulvae. Patient complains of weakness of bladder muscles and tone of bladder neck. Haematuria or high coloured urine. Urethral discharge if examined will confirm the disease.

Picric acid lady has signs of great degeneration of spinal cord with prostration, weakness and pain in back. Burning heat in spine. Headache generally begins with sunrise and the intensity increases with the day and is better by sleep at night. Extreme prostration after headache and also after sexual excitement. Sour eructations and nausea in the morning. Pains and loss of power of lower limbs with trembling and numbness.

Patient is much tired after least exertion. Brainfag. Lack of will power. Dislikes to work. Dementia with prostration. Lady sits quietly and listens to others as she is not in a position to think. The weakness of body and mind is marked characteristic of Picric acid lady. She is very sensitive to wet weather.

MODALITIES :

< Slightest exertion, mental work, wet weather, daytime, hot weather.

> From cold air, washing the parts with cold water, tight bandages.

2.2.3 COLLINSONIA

It acts predominantly on the inflamed vagina caused due to dysmenorrhoea and haemorrhoids resulting from chronic constipation. There is prolapse of external genitalia and pruritus. Patient is constipated and has to strain much for defecation. This causes excessive blood flow to vulval region resulting in congestion and redness of the parts with hyperaesthesia. Any infection of genitourinary tract or local skin lesion like psoriasis, eczema, fungal infections may result in secondary infection. The discharges from the lesion are acrid and foetid which irritate the parts.

Pelvic and portal congestion due to obstinate constipation is well marked in this remedy. This obstinate constipation results in haemorrhoids, bleeding per rectum and inflammation of genital tract. She has dull frontal headache. Yellowish white coating on tongue with bitter taste in mouth. She complains of cramp-like pain in stomach with nausea. Stool passes in lumps with great straining. Sharp, cutting pains in rectum. Sometimes constipation alternates with loose motions.

MODALITIES :

< From emotion, mental exertion and excitement, cold weather, cold applications, cold in general.

> Warmth in general, covering, rest.

2.2.4 MEZEREUM

Mezereum patient shows typical psoric manifestations like uncleanliness, unhygienic habits and bad clothing. Tight clothings, improper use of contraceptives and masturbation provoke the condition. Eruptions on the vulval region probably due to the suppression of eczema or skin diseases like psoriasis. Severe violent itching of the parts which makes the patient nervous and restless. Vesicular eruptions form thick, chalk-like white crusts, with violent itching and discharge of pus. Thick leucorrhoea like albumin, corroding in nature. She becomes the victim of hypochromic anaemia, deficiency of vitamin B complex or vitamin A. There is intense burning in tongue, extending to stomach with chronic gastritis. Nausea, vomiting coffee-ground material in gastric ulcer.

Patient is sad and melancholic. Mental symptoms are due to suppression of skin diseases. She has very weak memory. Due to intense itching the patient is very much restless and confused. Cannot answer the questions correctly and immediately. Has to think over the question. Nervous temperament.

MODALITIES :

< Cold air, warm food, warm drinks, up to midnight, in the evening, touch and movement.

> Open air.

2.2.5 BOVISTA

Eruptions and skin lesions are seen on various parts of the body including the genitalia. Eruptions like eczema on the vulval region is due to allergic reaction to fumes of charcoal. Lady complains of diarrhoea before and during menses. Voluptuous sensation. Acrid leucorrhoea which is thick, tough and greenish. She cannot bear tight clothings which causes irritation to vulval region. Intense soreness of the genitalia and pubic region during menses. Ovarian cysts are well marked in Bovista lady. Dull, bruised headache with stammering speech. She has a funny sensation as if there is a lump of ice in stomach. Cannot bear the tight clothing around the abdomen. Abdominal colic with high coloured urine. Relieved by eating indicates Bovista.

Patient is awkward and drops things from hands. She has sensation as if everything is enlarged. She is very sensitive to external impression.

MODALITIES :

< By tight clothing, touch.

> Open air, loose clothings around the waist.

2.2.6 GRAPHITES

Very useful remedy for skin eruptions which manifest typical psoric character. All types of skin eruptions on vulva are seen. These eruptions are always dry with intense itching. Sometimes the skin is inflamed causing local dermatitis. Cracked skin around the vulva. Erysipelas or eczema around the genitalia leads to violent itching. She scratches that local lesion and then the skin gets peeled off. So the skin becomes sore, inflamed and it bleeds. Thus the pruritus vulva of Graphites lady is solely due to the skin eruptions. Profuse sweating in the genital region.

Marked acuteness when any symptom appears or disappears. Coldness all over the body, especially in spots. Catarrhal condition of eyes, ears etc. with occipital headache. Daytime diarrhoea and nocturnal cough with hoarseness of voice.

Patient is dazed and very much confused; various imaginations. Patient imagines that she is going to die very soon. Everything looks double. During feverish delirium considers herself double and imagines some strange person near her. Sensation of coldness everywhere in the body.

MODALITIES :

< Before thunder storm, damp weather, mental work, change of season.

> Dry weather, warmth in general.

2.2.7 KALI CARBONICUM

The hormonal imbalance and the recurrent trauma to the genital tract due to miscarriage, deliveries and episiotomy after parturition may become the cause of pruritus vulvae. Cutting pain in abdomen after miscarriage. Pains traverse through left labium which extends through abdomen to chest. This remedy is well indicated in pruritus vulvae especially after parturition. Uterine haemorrhage which is constant and the flow is copious. Violent backache is always associated with pruritus, relieved by sitting and hard pressure.

Kali. carb lady has desire for sweets with flatulency. She has feeling of lump in the pit of stomach and has constant feeling as if stomach were full of water. She has to wake up several times at night to pass the urine. Sense of pressure on bladder before urine comes. Pain in left hypochondriac region and she has to turn to right side before she wakes up.

Very irritable and alternating moods. Despondent and full of fear and imaginations. She has strong feeling of the bed sinking down. Wants company, somebody to be with her all the time. She is very much sensitive to noise, pain and touch.

MODALITIES :

< In the morning, lying on left side, after coition, in cold climate.

> In warm weather, during daytime, while moving about, in the company.

Other useful remedies for pruritus vulvae are

1) AMBRA GRISEA
2) CANTHARIS
3) HELONIAS
4) RADIUM
5) SULPHUR

****

CHAPTER 3

DISEASES OF VAGINA

TOPIC 1

ACUTE VAGINITIS

3.1.1 HYDRASTIS

Vaginitis from excoriation and erosion of the cervix. The vaginal mucous membrane is inflamed and is very much sensitive. Cannot bear the touch. There is acrid, corroding leucorrhoea which is more after menses. Due to the primary infection inflammation sets in, which then ascends upwards causing finally pelvic inflammatory disease. The pains are of dragging type, dull, which give the sense of stiffness especially across the lumbar region. The pains are so severe that she has to take support of her hands while getting up from sitting position. Pruritus vulva is associated with acute vaginitis.

Hydrastis acts specially on all the mucous membranes, relaxing them and thus ultimately producing thick, yellowish, ropy secretions. Headache in frontal region, associated with constipation. Tongue is white, swollen and large, shows imprints of teeth. Sore feeling in stomach with weak digestion. Bitter taste in mouth. Gastritis, ulcers and cancer with pulsation in epigastrium. Dull dragging in right groin. Fissures around anus, prolapse of rectum. Haemorrhoids, even a light flow exhausts with contractions and spasms. Skin eruptions like variola. Profuse perspiration and unhealthy skin. Ulcers and lupus are well marked.

Patient is sad and depressed, cannot concentrate on her work because of physical disability, mental diversion. Thus commits mistakes in her daily work. Patient thinks that her disease is dreadful and she is going to die of this disease. She feels death is more preferable than the disease.

MODALITIES :

< Heat in general, warmth applications, heat of bed, thinking of the complaints.

> Cold applications, washing the parts by cold water, open air.

3.1.2 CANTHARIS

Vaginitis, secondary to the urinary tract infection. Patient gets urinary tract infection and as the parts are very near in females, infection readily travels to vagina. Thus when the patient complains of burning micturition and relevant symptoms of urinary tract infection with vaginitis, Cantharis should be thought of. Infectious vaginitis, can be treated well by this remedy. There is persistent purulent discharge, at times blood-stained, per vagina. Pruritus, pains and soreness in vulva is very common. Dysuria, passing of urine is a troublesome procedure.

Patient is pale, wretched, deathly appearance. Multiple vesicles on face. Pain and dryness in throat. Bloody mucus at stool with burning in anal region. Bleeding piles are well treated by Cantharis. There is sense of constriction of chest which arrests the breathing. Pains from hips to feet. Sciatica. Pains more on bending backwards.

Patient has furious delirium. Anxiety and restlessness result in rage. Crying, barking. Patient constantly attempts to do something. Fiery sexual desire. Sudden loss of conciousness with red face.

MODALITIES:

< Touch, while urinating, drinking cold water.

> Rubbing the parts

3.1.3 APIS MELLIFICA

Acts on vaginal tissues; which are oedematous and puffy, due to diseased condition. There is swelling of vulva, labia with stinging type of pains. Soreness with intolerance of heat. Touch causes intense pain. There is sense of tightness and bearing down as if menses would appear. Pains are more during day-time, worse by heat. Oophoritis, right ovary is more painful. Menses are suppressed. Inflammation of the endometrial lining of the uterus. The cystic swelling of ovary gets infected. Inflammation of the fallopian tube which suppresses the menstruation in young girls, profuse intermenstrual bleeding with heaviness in the abdomen.

Patient is thirstless. This remedy has the power to antidote the poisonous effects of various insect bites. The patient does not like to be covered. Kicks off her own clothes. Complaints come suddenly, violently and spread rapidly. Oedematous swelling of throat which causes hoarseness of voice. Inflammation of liver and spleen, pain under the ribs, which spreads upwards. Abdomen is very sensitive to touch. Pitting type of oedema. Constipation is associated with congestion of head. Scanty urine passes in drops. She has to strain for urination. Urine is burning and is bloody. Inflammation of kidney, ureter, bladder and urethra. Oedematous swelling of urethral opening. Bag-like swelling of lower eyelid.

The patient is frightful, enraged and jealous from suppressed skin rash. She is sad and melancholic. Weeps without any cause or reason. Irritable.

MODALITIES :

< Sleep, hot things, touch, bandaging, clothings.

> Cold applications, open air.

3.1.4 KREOSOTE

Corrosive itching within the vulval area. Burning and swelling of labia. Due to vaginitis, there is violent itching in between labia and thighs. Infection causes leucorrhoea to appear. Vaginitis in postmenopausal ladies due to hormonal imbalance or exposure of vagina in vaginal prolapse. Postoperative vaginitis is common in this group, following usually vaginal repair operations. Leucorrhoea is yellow, acrid with odour of green corn. Worse between periods, haemorrhage after coition.

Dull pain in frontal part of head as if a board is pressing. Lips are red and bleeding. Nausea and vomiting of food several hours after eating. Abdomen is distended. Burning haemorrhoids; urine is offensive, which causes violent itching of vulva and vagina. Disturbed sleep with tossing. Itching of affected parts worse towards evening. Pain in calf muscles.

Music causes palpitation and weeping. Patient is in lost mood, therefore thoughts vanish. She is forgetful, stupid, peevish, and irritable. She wants many things but throws them away when given. Sensation as if the limbs are paralysed.

MODALITIES :

< Open air, while resting, cold in general, when lying, after menstruation.

> Warm application, motion, hot food.

3.1.5 THUJA

Vagina is very sensitive. Warty growths on the vulva and perineum. Patient has warts, condylomata on external genitalia. History of suppression of gonorrhoea. Profuse leucorrhoea which is thick and greenish. Infection sets in after the overgrowth and which then ascends to fallopian tubes and ovaries. Severe pain in left ovary and in left inguinal region. Menses are scanty and retarded. Dryness of the walls of vagina. There is polypoid growth on walls of vagina. Pains in the ovarian region are more during periods. Pains are more even after gentle touch and while walking. Profuse perspiration before menses. Coition is very painful.

Thuja has a specific antibacterial action, as in gonorrhoea. Typical sycotic pains, that is tearing in muscles and parts, is presented by patient as a concomitant symptom. Chronic abdominal discomfort such as distension of abdomen, gurgling sound, loss of appetite. Constipation, with violent rectal pains, stitching and burning pains in rectal region. Urethra is swollen and inflamed. Urinary stream splits and is short. Sensation of trickling after urinating. Dry hacking cough. Warts, carbuncles, ulcers especially in ano-genital region. Herpetic eruptions are well treated by this remedy.

Patient has fixed ideas. Sensation as if strange person were at her side, as if soul and body were separated, as if something alive in abdomen and so on.

Vomiting; chronic diarrhoea alternates with constipation and stools are jelly-like. Menses are either early or late and metrorrhagia at the time of climacteric.

Patient is hysterical and very much indifferent. Weeping disposition, cannot talk without weeping. She is sad and gentle. Mind is weak and dull. Behaves strangely and does strange things. Fear of ghosts. She thinks that something bad will happen. Dread of solitude yet she is worse in company.

MODALITIES :

< Damp wet weather, in the evening, washing, after laundry work.

> Hard pressure, warmth, cold bathing, after sleep.

3.1.6 SENECIO AUREUS

It is an indicated drug for acute inflammation of vagina with burning and intense pain. These pains are like that of labour pains. Vagina is dry and hot. Dragging pains, itching makes her embarrassed. Menses are retarded or suppressed. Vaginitis after the use of IUCDs, functional amenorrhoea in young girls. Backache. Many a time vaginitis is secondary to urinary tract infection. Pains in the region of ovary and around the umbilicus.

This pain spreads all over the abdomen. Better after passing stools. Acute inflammation of upper respiratory tract, with laboured breathing.

She has inability to fix the mind on one subject. Despondent and nervous. Vaginitis makes her irritable. Great drowsiness and unpleasant dreams. Nervousness and sleeplessness.

MODALITIES :

< Warmth in general, touch.

> Washing parts by cold water, rest.

Other important remedies for vaginitis are

1) GELSEMIUM
2) BELLADONNA
3) ARNICA MONTANA
4) KALI-CARB.
5) MERC-COR.

========

TOPIC 2

VAGINISMUS

3.2.1 COCCULUS INDICUS

Spasmodic pains due to contraction of the pelvic floor muscles, often associated with pain of gluteal muscles. Patient becomes opisthotonic whenever coitus is attempted. Suitable in newly married girls who are very sensitive. Parts are dry and inflamed. Leucorrhoea after menses. Injury and inflammation after the act of coition causes leucorrhoea. Intense pains with bruised feeling in back. Dysmenorrhoea - spasmodic type, with violent cramping pain at the time of menses.

Head is congested with pressing and throbbing pains. Neuralgic pains in the back and in perineum. Nausea with no desire to eat. The smell of food or just the thought of food makes the patient gag and she nauseates. Paralytic condition of oesophagus and intestinal canal. Spasms of muscles of stomach.

All the mental activities are depressed due to sleep. Sensation as if time passes very quickly. Mind is confused, not able to think. Feels that some unusual thing is going to happen. Fear of death.

MODALITIES :

< Motion, due to anxiety, grief, loss of sleep, after exertion, exposure to cold.

> Rest.

3.2.2 ARNICA

Vaginismus after forceful coition. Sore, lame and bruised

pains in vagina. Bleeding from uterus and vaginal wall after mechanical injury or after coition. Retention of urine after mechanical injury. The parts are very sensitive to touch.

Extravasation of blood from the capillaries, sore and bruised feeling all over the body. This drug has the power to control all the bad effects of injuries. It also controls all inflammatory conditions of the body. The patient is hypersensitive and does not want to be touched or approached.

Patient is sad, melancholic, irritable and fearful. Imagines that she has got some dreadful disease and death is near to her.

MODALITIES :

< Touch, rest, damp, cold.

> When left alone.

3.2.3 THUJA OCCIDENTALIS

Patients are prone to get uro-genital infections as there is history of suppression of sycotic dyscrasia. Patient complains of intense sensitiveness of the vagina. Any touch or the attempt of coition provokes the perineal muscles and the vaginal walls to go into a spasm, causing severe painful condition. Thus it is useful also in dyspareunia. Increased frequency of micturition. Severe cutting pains in vagina. Profuse leucorrhoea, thick and greenish discharge from the vagina. There are warty growths on vaginal walls. These also cause lot of disturbances to the patient. Sometimes these bleed on touch. Pains in ovarian region, especially of left ovary.

The patient has rapid exhaustion and emaciation. Tearing pains in muscles and also in joints. These typical pains are termed as "sycotic pains". Patient complains of chronic inflammatory condition and consequently the suppurative stage. The common affected parts are eyes, ears, gums, nose etc. The discharges are greenish, thick and offensive.

Mentally patient is idiotic and sluggish. Has fixed ideas in mind. Emotional sensitiveness. Patient takes some strange notions in her mind and keeps on thinking.

MODALITIES :

< At night, damp wet weather, cold air, touch, heat of bed.

> Open air.

3.2.4 PLATINA

This remedy is indicated in patients who complain of hypersensitiveness of parts. There is tingling numbness and coldness of the genital parts. Hyperaesthesia of the genitals. Genitals are very sensitive to touch. Parts go into spasm when touched or sometimes during coition she faints. Nymphomania marked in young girls. Ovaries are hypersensitive with burning sensation. This remedy also acts well in condition of pruritus vulvae. Abnormal sexual appetite is seen in this remedy.

Menorrhagia or metrorrhagia is the concomitant symptom of vaginismus in Platina. Menses are profuse and early. Blood is black and coagulated. Cramp-like pains with paralytic weakness of the extremities. There is sense of constriction in the limbs. They are cold and stiff.

Mental symptoms of Platina lady alternate with physical symptoms. She becomes a victim of the disease due to disappointment, fright, uterine troubles, excitement and sexual excesses. Sad and weeping mood alternates with joy and happiness. Becomes serious on silly matters. Many times it is observed that these mental symptoms are intermingled with the uterine and sexual symptoms.

MODALITIES :

< On sitting and standing, in the evening.

> Walking, open air.

3.2.5 MUREX

Murex ladies are very conscious about the genital parts. Pulsations in the cervical os. Exhausted and excited easily. There is a feeling of hard pressing upon the parts. Sore spots in the pelvic organs. This soreness is very much strong while sitting. There is intense pain in the left ovarian region and also in left breast. Nymphomania is predominant. Sore pain in the uterine region. Uterus is bulky and indurated. Severe tenesmus in the pelvic region which ascends to left breast. Patient shows the signs of chronic endometritis with dysmenorrhoea. Uterine displacement and flaccid uterine supports. Thus there is prolapse of uterus. Patient has to cross her legs to prevent something protruding out. Profuse leucorrhoea which is bloody and green. Sharp cutting pains in the sacral region.

There is sinking and all-gone sensation in stomach. Patient has great hunger and she has to eat frequently. Increased frequency of urination at night. Urge to pass urine.

Patient is sad and anguished. There is great anxiety about work and the things which will happen in the future. Patient has dreadful thoughts.

MODALITIES :

< Least touch, noise.

> Open air, rest.

3.2.6 IGNATIA

There are nervous and hysterical factors which play a great role in the patient to arrive at this condition. Patient is very much excited and is melancholic. Thus she wants to remain isolated. As she is nervous and apprehensive, there is lack of vaginal secretion which causes dryness and vaginismus. Ignatia acts well both in psychological vaginismus and perineal vaginismus. Patient has complete aversion to sexual performance. Thus the act of coition causes painful spasm of perineal muscles. There is spasmodic pain in the uterine region and in stomach. Patient shows sexual frigidity. This frigidity in Ignatia lady might be due to disappointment in the past and suppression of grief.

Ignatia lady has marked hyperaesthesia of all the senses. Thus there is a tendency to clonic spasm. There is feeling of lump in vagina and also in the throat. Sour eructations. Empty sensation or all-gone feeling in stomach with cramps in stomach. There is dry, spasmodic cough with little expectoration. Menses are black which are too early and too profuse. Jerking pains in the limbs. Sleep is very light.

Patient is mentally sad with long involuntary sighing. There is changeable mood and she sits brooding silently. Melancholic, sad and tearful. Patient is not at all communicable. Mental symptoms follow suppression of grief and disappointment.

MODALITIES :

< In the morning, open air, after meals and warm applications externally.

> By changing the position, while eating.

3.2.7 CAULOPHYLLUM

Patient has lack of tonicity of the pelvic organs. The supports of the uterus and the ovaries are relaxed due to multiple deliveries, where the labour pains are deficient and the patient has to strain much to deliver the baby. Extraordinary rigid os is seen only in Caulophyllum, therefore act of coition causes severe spasmodic pains in the uterine region which fly in all directions. Menses are too profuse with discharges of dark, clotted blood. Patient gives the history of habitual abortions due to uterine debility. Pricking pains in the cervical region during the act of coition.

Caulophyllum is the remedy frequently used for severe drawing and erratic pains and stiffness in small joints, fingers and toes. There are piercing pains in the wrist joint and cutting pains in fingers on clenching; cannot keep a particular position for longer time. Patient complains of discolouration of the skin with menstrual and uterine disorders.

Patient is hysterical. Great apprehension and fear of coitus due to the pains during the act. She tries to avoid it. She is restless due to pains.

MODALITIES :

< Cold, open air.

> By emssion of flatus.

Other important remedies for vaginismus are

1. BELLADONNA
2. STAPHYSAGRIA
3. BERBERIS VULGARIS
4. CARBO VEG.
5. TARENTULA HISPANIA

****

CHAPTER 4

DISEASES OF CERVIX

TOPIC 1

ENDOCERVICITIS

4.1.1 THUJA OCCIDENTALIS

It is a great, deep-acting remedy, indicated for the chronic endocervicitis usually due to suppressed gonorrhoea. Violent pain in the cervical canal with intense pruritus. Menses are offensive, profuse, dark and clotted, stains are difficult to washout. Whole cervical canal is sensitive due to chronic endocervicitis. Leucorrhoea, which is thin, acrid and excoriating with fishy odour.

There is high grade fever secondary to infection with low backache. Patient wants to be fanned all the time. Chills up and down the back. Tongue thickly coated, brown and white. Oppressed breathing.

Patient has weak memory. Loses thread of the conversation. Patient has weeping mood and cannot narrate the symptoms without weeping. Time passes too slowly. Patient has lost all hopes of recovery. Patient is nervous and restless Melancholy with suicidal thoughts.

MODALITIES :

< On thinking of her ailments, from sunrise to sunset, heat in general.

> Damp wet weather, lying on stomach.

4.1.2 HEPAR SULPH

Discharges of blood and mucus from the uterus after labour or abortion when secondary infection sets in. The whole cervical canal is affected with tendency to suppurate. There are multiple small papules on the endocervical region, which ultimately turns into pustules. There is high grade fever when papules turn into pustules. Menses are late and scanty.

Abscesses of labia with great sensitiveness due to chronic suppurative condition. The leucorrhoea is very offensive. Leucorrhoea smells like old cheese.

Patient has yellowish complexion. Middle of lower lip is cracked. There is intense burning in stomach with pressure and heaviness after slight meal. Patient voids small quantity of urine drop by drop as the muscles of bladder go weak.

Aphonia; cough when exposed to dry cold wind. Hoarseness of voice. Wheezing in dry cold air. Abscess, suppurating glands are hypersensitive. There is great sensitiveness to slightest touch. Putrid ulcer.

Anguish in the evening and at night, with suicidal thoughts crowding in mind. Trifles factors irritate her mind. Patient is very much sad and dejected. Ferocious, she speaks very rapidly. Hasty in all work.

MODALITIES :

< Dry cold wind, cold air, touch.

> Damp wet weather, warmth, wrapping the parts.

4.1.3 SULPHURIC ACID

This remedy acts well especially in the patients of climacteric age group. Due to prolapse of the uterus, secondary infection sets in and this infection is transmitted in the cervical canal. Endocervicitis is common in child bearing age due to transmitted infections like Neisseria gonorrhoeae, Chlamydia trachomatis, Mycoplasma species and also pyogenic infections during childbirth, abortion and instrumentation.

Chronic endocervicitis with mucous discharge, which is acrid and burning. Leucorrhoea associated with bloody mucus calls for this remedy.

Heartburn with sour eructations. Nausea with chilliness. Menses are early and profuse. Right-sided neuralgia with throbbing pain in left orbital region is well treated by this remedy. Pain in the occipital region (right side) relieved by holding the hands near head. Gums bleed easily. Writer's cramp with history of lead poisoning.

Patient is fearful and very restless. Wants to do everything very soon. Very impatient, wants to hurry in all matters. Reluctant to answer questions.

MODALITIES :

< Excess of heat and cold, forenoon and evening.

> Warmth in general and lying down.

4.1.4 ARSENIC ALBUM

Oedematous swelling of the genitalia. Syphilitic ulcers of the endocervical region with burning and stinging pains. Patient complains of dryness and itching of vagina due to inflammatory condition of endocervical mucous membrane. There is excoriating discharge which is thick and acrid. Chronic inflammation many times leads to malignancy of cervix. Hypertrophy and elongation of cervix with everted round cell infiltration around endocervical glands and in the cervical stroma. Endocervical region shows picture of proliferation of columnar epithelial cells.

Patient complains dryness of mouth with unquenchable thirst. Yet she takes little quantity of cold water, just to moisten dry mouth. Stomach is very sensitive to touch with great burning which is relieved by warm drink. Catarrhal condition of respiratory tract with hoarsenss of voice and burning. Dry, scaly eruptions of skin, burn like fire. Syphilitic ulcers on genitals.

Mentally patient is very much restless, anxious and there is suicidal tendency. Great fear of death. Doesn't want to meet people. Patient is fastidious. She wants everything to be kept in order, neat and clean.

MODALITIES :

< Cold, cold food, cold drinks, over-ripe fruits, exertion, midday, midnight.

> Warmth or heat in general, hot drinks, rest.

4.1.5 HYDRASTIS

The mucous membrane of the cervical canal is affected. There is a sense of relaxation. Secretions are thick, yellowish and ropy. Catarrh of endocervical canal, vagina is excoriated. Burning at vulval region. Leucorrhoea is more after menstruation. Pruritus vulvae. There are evidences of chronic inflammation with round cell infiltration around endocervical glands.

Endocervicitis is many a time associated with metrorrhagia or intermenstrual bleeding. Pains in back and in lumbar region. Weakness of the muscles of back. Gastroduodenal catarrh. Patient complains of chronic constipation. Follicular pharyngitis. Skin is excoriated, ulcerated, which is worse from heat in general.

Patient is very sad and depressed. She is sure that she is going to die, the death is certain due to long-lasting disease. Patient is discouraged due to prolonged sufferings hence disgusted and cannot concentrate her mind on a particular work.

MODALITIES :

< Warmth in general, heat of bed, movement.

> Rest, open air, cold in general.

4.1.6 MERCURIUS SOL

Chronic cervicitis in Merc. sol. ladies is commonly localised in the endocervical mucosa; with chronic inflammatory lesion in the surrounding fibromuscular structure of cervix. Chronic inflammation due to suppressed sexually transmitted infections and diseases. Burning, stinging, tearing and cutting pains in ovarian region. Parts are sore due to excoriating leucorrhoea which is pale, acrid, and makes the parts inflamed and sore. Formation of multiple boils in and around the genitalia.

Menses are profuse with abdominal pain. Sensation of rawness in parts. Stinging pain in the ovarian region. Skin is almost constantly moist. Ulcers are irregular in shape, edges are undefined. Sweetish metallic taste in the mouth, salivary secretions are greatly increased. Vertigo when lying on back. Inflammatory condition of the respiratory tract. History of habitual abortion. Rheumatic affections of the joints. Ulcers or abscesses on legs. Cold perspiration on lower extremities.

Patient is depressed and very slow in answering the questions. Loss of memory or will power. Patient thinks that she will lose reason.

MODALITIES:

< Night; in damp wet weather; change of season; after perspiration.

> Rest, open air, sitting position.

4.1.7 NITRIC ACID

Soreness of the external genital organs with multiple ulcers in the endocervical region. Leucorrhoea is associated with inflammation of the cervical canal, cervix looks angry red with sloughs on it. Menses are early, profuse, like muddy water. Uterine haemorrhage due to ascending infection. Stitching in vagina and in cervical region. Pains traversing to hips, back of thighs.

Great hunger with sweetish taste in mouth. Patient has to strain much but passes little stools. Rectum feels torn. Scanty, dark urine which is offensive in nature. Sensation of band around the head; foetid foot sweat, causing soreness of toes with stitching pains in toes.

MODALITIES :

< In the evening, at night, cold climate and also hot weather.

> While riding in carriage.

Other important remedies for endocervicitis are

1. LYCOPODIUM
2. SEPIA
3. KREOSOTE
4. CARBOLIC ACID
5. CARBO ANIMALIS

===========

TOPIC 2

CERVICAL EROSION

4.2.1 ARSENICUM ALBUM

On cervical mucous membranes it causes ulceration and later on gangrene. There is cervical erosion which manifests profuse menorrhagia, leucorrhoea and typical internal burning of Arsenic. There is intense burning in ovarian region. Leucorrhoea is also acrid, offensive, burns the parts, thin and watery, having fetid or cadaveric smell. Pains are like from red hot wires. Vagina is dry with intense burning, itches much. Due to proliferation of columnar epithelium, it gets folded and forms papillary projections on granulation tissue, which are obviously seen in chronic cervicitis. Oedematous swelling of genitalia. Burning and stitching pains in the cervical region. Dryness and itching of the vagina. Copious, thin, whitish and excoriating discharges from vagina. Menstrual flow is acrid and offensive. Sexually transmitted diseases cause ulcers on cervix; like syphilitic ulcers, which then turn into chronic cervical erosion.

Periodical headache can be seen, which is of psoric or syphilitic character. Gastric troubles due to taking cold things, spoiled food and over-ripened fruits. She complains of recurrent catarrhal condition of respiratory tract with hoarseness of voice and sense of burning. Mouth is dry and patient drinks sip by sip to moisten her mouth. Easily exhausted after slight work or trouble. Cannot bear sight or smell of food, it nauseates her. Except of the head, all pains are relieved by warmth. Patient is cachectic and has low vitality. Periodicity is well marked in Arsenic patients. Symptoms are worse at midday and midnight. Patient is so much exhausted that she is unable to turn in the bed.

MODALITIES :

< Midday andmid night, from cold and cold drinks, alcohol, wet weather.

> Warm drinks, rest, elevation of head, heat in general.

4.2.2 VESPA CRABRO

Acquired erosion around the external os is well treated by this remedy. The squamous epithelium regrows towards the external os, replacing the columnar epithelium which is made to atrophy and subsequently disappears. There is proliferation alternately of basal cells and columnar epithelium.

Left ovary is markedly affected. Menstruation preceded by depression, pain, pressure and constipation. Increased frequency of micturition. Burning in urethra. Sacral pains extending to back. Erosion of the external os, which is angry red with discharges, which are foul smelling. Patient is dizzy with sense of fainting. Perspiration of the parts with itching. Burning micturition with itching in urethra.

Patient is depressed and there is sense of pressure on vertex.

MODALITIES :

Itching and soreness is ameliorated by bathing with vinegar.

4.2.3 AURUM METALLICUM

Cervical erosion due to prolapse of the uterus. In the early stage of prolapse, there is establishment of cervicitis, desquamation and shedding of epithelium around the external os occurs. The affected area around the external os, on the portio vaginalis, shows the covering of columnar epithelium with the formation of new glands. There may be backache at the lower part of sacrum with frequency of micturition and dysuria. This is probably due to spread of infection around the bladder wall. Pruritus vulvae is always present with Aurum metallicum.

Patient complains of great sensitiveness of vagina with

vaginismus. Dropsy of lower limbs. Paralytic tearing pains in joints. Knees are weak. Patient is sleepless, if sleeps, has frightful dreams. Extreme photophobia. Appetite and thirst is increased. Pain in the right hypochondriac region. Patient has profound despondency with increased blood pressure. Patient is disgusted in life and thinks of suicide. She always talks of committing suicide. Great fear of death. Mental derangements with syphilitic characters. Cannot do things fast enough. Patient is confused and excited.

MODALITIES :

- < In cold weather, when getting cold, winter season, from sunset to sunrise.
- > Warmth in general, sunrise to sunset.

4.2.4 HYDRASTIS

Hydrastis acts specially on the mucous membrane of the cervix where there are thick, yellowish ropy secretions due to cervical erosion. There is proliferation of columnar epithelium which gets folded and forms papillary projections. On the surface there are pseudoglands or crypts formed in between the papillae. The reddened area on the portio vaginalis around the external os is present. Constant bathing of epithelium by irritating discharges. The denuded area is being covered by the columnar epithelium of endocervix. The superficial parts of the cervix, near the cervical os is formed by epithelial lining. Due to erosion, excoriation of cervix is seen.

Leucorrhoea, worse after menses. Acrid and corroding discharges. Menorrhagia, blood is dark and frank. Pruritus vulvae with profuse leucorrhoea. Sexual excitement with leucorrhoea. Hydrastis lady also has tumour of breast with retracted nipples. Follicular pharyngitis with raw, smarting, excoriating sensation. Hacking of yellow, tenacious mucus. Gastro-duodenal catarrh. Liver region is tender. Sometimes associated with gall-stones. Dull, heavy, dragging pain across lumbar region especially during bleeding per-vagina.

Patient is depressed and she thinks that she will definitely die due to this disease and she desires it.

CERVICAL EROSION

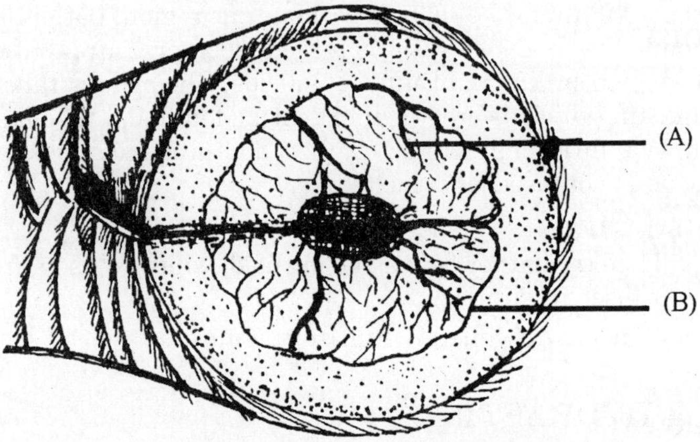

Cervical erosion : (papillary type)

(A) Naboth's Follicles (B) Granular surface

4.2.5 SULPHURIC ACID

Erosion of the cervix in those who have crossed menopause. Red granular surface with well defined margins are visible on cervical os. Both lips of cervix are commonly involved. The surface is seen smeared with white discharge. The surface of portio vaginalis shows multiple small, pearly white, nodular elevations. Metrorrhagia, especially after sexual intercourse is common feature of Sulphuric acid patient.

Patients are commonly debilitated with right-sided neuralgia. Cramps and compressive pains in the arms. Writer's cramps. Weak feeling with dragging into hips. Hernia would protrude especially of left side. Early and profuse menstruation. Ladies of multiparity and of middle age complain of erosion of cervix which bleeds very easily. Acrid and burning leucorrhoea often with mucous membrane.

Patient is fearful, cannot concentrate her mind. Impatient. Unwilling to answer questions. Makes hurry in all work. Wants everything very soon.

MODALITIES :

< Excess of heat or cold, in forenoon or in the evening.

> From warmth in general and wrapping the parts.

4.2.6 CONIUM

Induration of the cervical os with metrorrhagia. Menses are scanty and suppressed. Chronic ill-health with muscular pains which are of stitching and tearing type.

Usually a follicular erosion which is velvety or small, hard. Cervix is bulky, firm and elongated with lacerations, especially at the lateral angles. Vaginal smear and cervical scrape prove the diagnosis. The endocervix and cervical stroma shows the picture of chronic inflammation, round cell infiltration and fibrosis of inflammatory type.

Cancerous condition of stomach, ulceration of stomach. Pinching, stitching, cutting, cramping and colicky pain in the abdomen. The bowels are constipated due to paralytic weakness of the rectum. Ovaries and uterus are enlarged and indurated. Burning, stinging and tearing pain in the external os. Menses are scanty and suppressed. Throbbing, tearing and burning pain in uterus. Mammary glands are sore and inflamed.

Patient is greatly debilitated and tired. Not in a position to make any mental efforts nor she is able to think. Weakness of mind with weak memory. Hates people. Excitement makes the patient weak and sad. Patient is confused and loses the thoughts.

MODALITIES :

< Cold, bad effects of injury, suppression of desire, movements in the bed.

> Motion, by hanging the limbs down the bed.

4.2.7 CARBO ANIMALIS

Ulcers especially on the lower lip of the cervix with metastatic infection. Chronic endocervical infection. Chronic endocervicitis with mucous discharges infect the cervical os and thus there is cervical erosion. Patient complains of persistent white discharge which is thick in nature, sometimes muco-purulent. There may be backache at lower part of sacrum. Metrorrhagia. Nausea worse at night. Lochia offensive, menses too early, frequent, long-lasting, followed by great exhaustion. Severe stitching pains in the cervical region.

Spongy ulcers on the skin with copper coloured eruptions. Pain in the coccyx, burns when touched. Even eating tires the patient. Patient has scrofulous and venous constitution. Glands are indurated. Weakness of nursing women. Headache with sensation as if head were blown to pieces. Rush of blood with confusion.

Patient desires to be alone. She is sad and reflective. Patient has inclination to avoid conversation. She is very much anxious at night.

MODALITIES :

< Loss of animal fluid.

> Open air, rest in bed.

Other useful remedies for cervical erosion are

1) SEPIA
2) MUREX
3) PHYTOLACCA
4) KREOSOTE
5) KALI ARS.
6) HYDROCOTYLE

===========

Topic 3

CERVICAL POLYP

4.3.1 CALCAREA FLUORICA

A pedunculated hard growth arising from the membrane of cervix can be well treated by this remedy. History of sexually transmitted diseases or suppression of syphilis may be the fundamental cause. These patients have the tendency for overgrowth. Patient complains of pains of cutting type in the cervical region and also in genitals. Bleeds on touch, which is dark red in colour, pain in back extending to the sacrum worse by rest and better by continuous motion and by warm application.

Inflammation of cervical os; cutting pain in the region of liver, nausea and vomiting of undigested food. Painful bleeding piles can be well treated by this remedy. Bowels are constipated. Hacking and spasmodic cough with hoarseness of voice associated with breathlessness. Patient is chilly and is sensitive to cold air. Induration and stony hard swelling of glands.

Patient is sad, and she has depressed mood. Melancholic temperament. Due to disease she is miserable and confused.

MODALITIES :

< Cold, cold air; cold applications, change of weather and rest.

> Warmth in general; continuous movement, motion.

4.3.2 HYDROCOTYLE

This remedy is indicated in the condition where inflammation or cellular proliferation of cervical tissues takes place, so as to form the cervical polyp. Hypertrophy or induration of cells of cervix takes place. Prominent and chief action of this remedy is on connective tissues of the cervix. Cervical growth sometimes protrude into the vagina which bleeds on touch. Profuse leucorrhoea with burning and itching in the vagina. Cervix is red. Dull pain in the region of ovary. There is ulceration of cervical mucous membrane with pruritus of vagina.

Skin is thickened and exfoliated. Profuse sweating all over the body with itching especially in the soles. Severe dull pain in nape of neck causes giddiness; patient cannot maintain up-right position. Pustules on the chest. Psoriasis, circular spots with scaly edges. Syphilitic skin manifestation. Useful for elephantiasis.

Patient is confused with sluggish movements. Lack of concentration.

4.3.3 THUJA OCCIDENTALIS

It is king of antisycotic remedies. Patient has the tendency to form an extra growth usually in genito-urinary tract. Cervical polyp is the common condition seen in patient who gives history of suppressed gonorrhoeal infection. Wart-like excrescences, fig-warts are seen in external genitalia, pedunculated, pale growth of cervical polyp is seen. Cervical erosion; catarrhal condition of mucous membrane of the cervical canal and vagina. Vagina is very sensitive. Due to infectious polypous growth, patient complaints of leucorrhoea which is thick greenish, with severe pains in ovarian region.

Neuralgic pains due to suppressed sycotic discharges or supressed gonorrhoea. Stitching pains start from the cervical region and extend to the back. She has severe pain in left ovary at the time of menses. Strong pungent smell of mouth especially when there is warty growth in the buccal cavity.

Mental symptoms are associated with the chief complaints. Typical fixed ideas of the particular lady can be heard from her. She thinks over the problem and makes her own conclusions. She thinks that she is pregnant and some thing alive is moving in the abdomen. Somebody is following her and is behind her and so on.

MODALITIES :

< At night, from heat of bed, from cold damp air.

> In open air.

4.3.4 SABINA

This is the remedy used in cervical polyp, which is associated with shooting pains from sacrum to pubis, and from vagina to uterus. Mucous polyp is well treated by this remedy. There is an overgrowth of the endometrium or endocervix. Excessive hormonal stimulation is an important factor for

CERVICAL POLYP

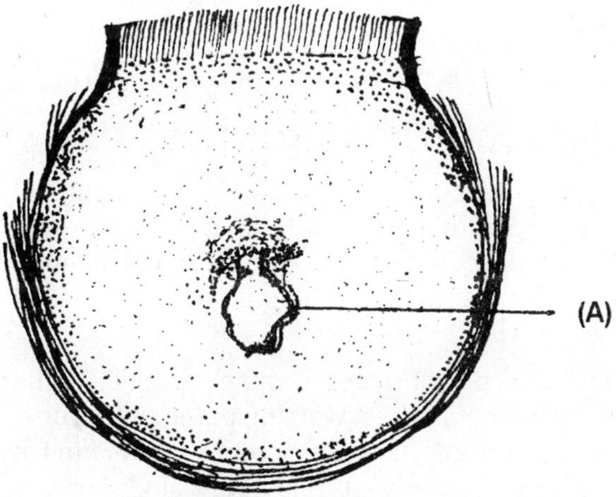

(A) Cervical mucous polyp

these types of overgrowths. These are small, size of a pea. Single or multiple, which bleed on touch.

Sabina is one of the important antihaemorrhagic remedy. This patient has tendency to bleed profusely, blood is bright red in colour. Pulsation all over the body with sense of fulness. Shooting pains from sacrum to pubis or from back to front in all menstrual disorders, or in case of cervical polyp. There is intense chill during the period of bleeding, which makes the patient lie down. Intermittent bleeding. Bleeding between the periods is the characteristic symptom of Sabina. Sexual desire is increased. History of suppression of sexually transmitted disease, result of this is the sycotic overgrowth. Burning and throbbing pains in urethra. Lancinating pain from pit of stomach across the back. Bruised pains on anterior portion of thighs. Fig-warts with intolerable itching and burning.

Patient is nervous due to the overgrowth and also due to sycotic miasm. Music is intolerable. Cannot concentrate her mind, confused.

MODALITIES :

< Least movement, motion, heat, warmth in general, warm room.

> In cool fresh air.

4.3.5 CALCAREA CARBONICA

Cervical polyps are bright red in colour, thin-walled and are usually pedunculated. These are soft and slippery. Endocervical polyp may show a typical epithelium or squamous metaplasia simulating malignancy. Tendency to reappear or relapse.

Patient gives history of headache, colic, chilliness and leucorrhoea before menses. Cutting pains in uterus before and during menstruation. Breasts become tender and hot before menses. Milky leucorrhoea. Tickling cough, troublesome at night. Free expectoration in the morning. Burning and soreness in the chest. Rheumatic pains. Cramps in calf muscles. Sour foot sweat; burning of soles, weakness of extremities. Abdomen is sensitive to slight pressure. Liver region is tender and sense of fullness in right hypochondriac region.

Patient is very apprehensive especially in the evening. She fears she will lose reason. Forgetful, confused, low spirited.

Little mental exertion produces head hot. Headache from mental worries. Aversion to work or exertion.

MODALITIES :

< From exertion, mental or physical; cold in every form, cold water, wet weather.

> Dry climate, dry weather.

4.3.6 FRAXINUS AMERICANA

This remedy acts well on overgrowths of uterus as well as cervix. Fibrous growth of the endocervix, which arises by process of extrusion from submucous lining. The tumour leaves the capsular bed and becomes pedunculated. The size may be moderate to large. It is usually pedunculated or very rarely sessile, lying in the vagina or in cervical os.

Depression with nervous restlessness, anxiety. Sensation of hot spot on top of head.

4.3.7 KALI IODIDE

Cervical polyp or subinvolution type of polyp. It has capsule of endometrium or endocervix from which the polyp gets the blood supply. The pedicle consists of the covering of mucuous membrane. Very rarely these polyps may show adenomyomatous structure. Large polyp gets ulcerated and infected subsequently.

Menses are late and profuse. During menstrual flow uterus feels as if squeezed. Due to infected cervical polyp there is leucorrhoea, which is corrosive in nature. Nasal discharge is profuse, acrid, hot and watery. Violent, throbbing headache, in temporals. Profuse watery, acrid coryza associated with cervical polyp serves as a sure guiding symptom.

Patient is harsh tempered, anxious and sad. She is very irritable as there is congestion to head, slightest noise causes lot of disturbances and irritation.

MODALITIES :

< Warm clothings, warm room, at night and damp wet weather.

> Open air, movement.

Other important remedies for cervical polyp are

1. CONIUM
2. SANGUINARIA
3. PHOSPHORUS
4. AURUM IODIDE
5. LACHESIS

============

TOPIC 4

CARCINOMA OF CERVIX

4.4.1 IODUM

Patient complains of induration and swelling of the cervix. The average age of the women is about 35 years. Cancerous growth due to hormonal imbalance and chronic irritation. There is atypical cellular proliferation from basal cell, part to almost full thickness of stratified squamous and columnar epithelium of cervix. The term dysplasia is used for the same.

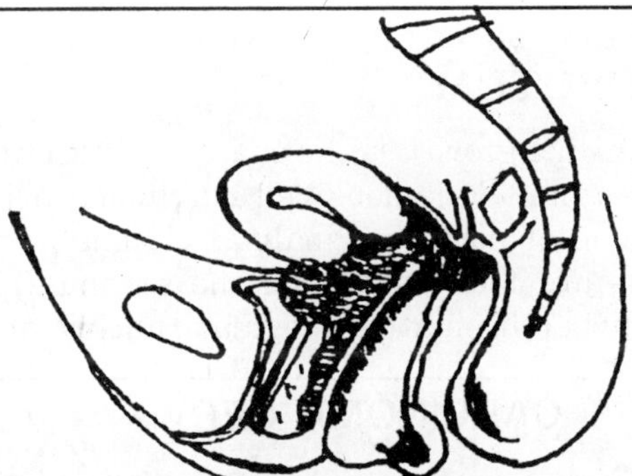

Stage IV : Ca. involved mucous wall of baldder & rectum

There is hypertrophy of cervical canal and cervical os. Due to secondary infection, there occura leucorrhoea, which is thick, slimy, bloody, acrid and excoriates the thighs. Induration and inflammation of the cervix. Acts better on grade I type of neoplasia where mild dysplasia takes place and slight changes have been observed in cervical glands. These cervical glands are hypertrophied and hard.

There is catarrhal inflammation of eyes with ulceration. Rapid metabolism. There is great appetite yet she loses flesh. Increased thirst. Patient is always better after eating. Great debility. The slightest effort induces perspiration. This remedy acts effectively on connective tissues. Constriction of larynx. Enlargement of the thyroid gland. Bleeding per rectum. Patient is constipated. Constipation alternates with diarrhoea. Menorrhagia, great weakness during irregular menses. Inflammation of the ovaries, i.e. oophoritis, wedge-like pain from ovary to uterus. Acrid leucorrhoea.

Mentally patient is anxious when quiet. She presents herself with anxiety and depression. There is sudden impulse to run and to do violence. Forgetful; must be busy. Fear of people. She has suicidal tendency.

MODALITIES :

< When quiet, in warm room.

> Walking, open air.

4.4.2 KREOSOTUM

Cauliflower-like growth is the characteristic or diagnostic feature of Kreosote. Squamous cell carcinoma arising from transitional zone of portio vaginalis. Columns of malignant epithelial cells are found invading the stroma. These cells show large hyperchromatic irregular nuclei and scanty

CARCINOMA CERVIX

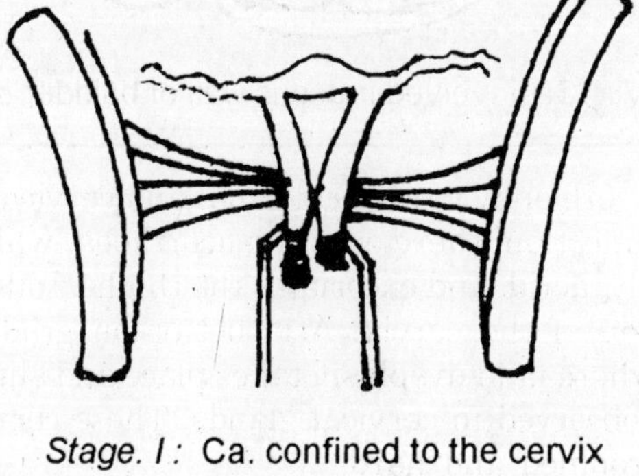

Stage. I : Ca. confined to the cervix

cytoplasm. There is irritation of overgrowth in vagina and in vulval region. Thus there is intense burning and itching of the parts. Due to secondary infection there is swelling and induration of labia and violent itching between labial folds.

Menorrhagia, irregular bleeding; postcoital bleeding or bleeding on straining or post-menopausal or intermenstrual bleeding. There is leucorrhoea which is yellow, acrid and with odour of green corn, worse between periods. Menses are too early and profuse.

Kreosotum lady presents with signs of rapid decomposition of fluids and secretions. Dull headache usually at the time of menses. Lips are dry and bleeding from cracks. Hoarseness with pain in larynx. Winter cough in post-menopausal ladies.

Patient is very sad. Especially music causes her lot of disturbances and palpitation. Thus mental disturbances result in vanishing of thoughts. She is stupid, forgetful and peevish with lot of mental irritation.

MODALITIES :

< In open air, cold in general, rest, when lying in bed, after menstruation.

> Warmth in general, movement.

4.4.3 NATRUM CARB

Induration of the cervix with sore pudenda. Severe sacral pains, radiating to the thighs, as lumbosacral nerve plexus is involved. After cervical biopsy columns of the malignant epithelial cells are found invading the stroma and the malignant cells show large, hyperchromatic, irregular nuclei. In naked eye examination, endocervical growth is seen where a papillary node appears in the cervical canal which gradually invades the cervical structure making the cervix barrel shaped. There is bearing down sensation and heaviness in cervix which is worse by sitting; better by moving. Menses are late and scanty, like meat washing. Leucorrhoeal discharge is offensive, irritating and preceded by colic.

Nat. carb. lady presents always with anaemia and prostration causing systemic changes. All the disturbances are caused due to sunstroke or heat of sun. Headache is also from heat of sun or from working under gaslight. She perspires very easily. Eruptions on toes and fingers. Increased venous filling. Nose shows pimples and other eruptions with constant coryza causing obstruction of nose. Nasal secretions are offensive. Patient has aversion to milk. Depressed after eating. Sudden urge to pass the stool. Milk causes loose motions. Patient complains of dry cough especially when she comes to warm room from outdoors.

Patient is unable to think. She has mental weakness with depression; worried and very sensitive to noise. She is sensitive to presence of certain individuals.

MODALITIES :

< By sitting, from music, heat of sun, mental exertion, change of weather.

> Movements.

4.4.4 CARBO ANIMALIS

This remedy has broken down or exhausted constitution. Old ladies with impaired circulation, low vitality. May present with past history of some debilitating diseases like tuberculosis. Early menstruation which is profuse. Exhausting menses. Burning pains down the thighs. Menstruates only in morning.

CARCINOMA CERVIX

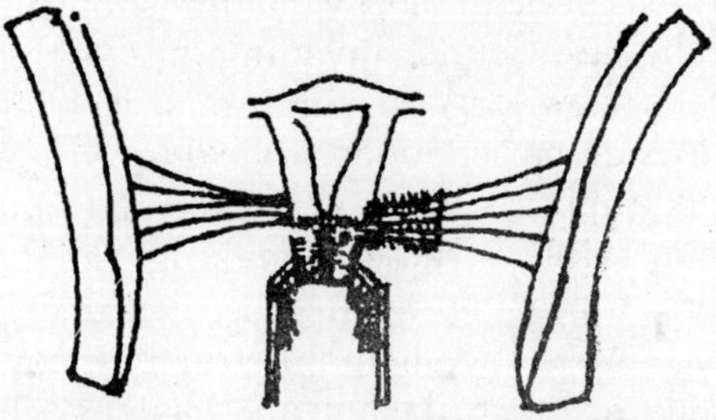

Stage. II : Ca. involves the vagina

She complains of profuse leucorrhoea with very much offensiveness. All-gone sensation in stomach during lactation.

Inflammation has tendency to go into chronicity and naturally it turns into malignant growths. The veins of the particular parts become tortuous and engorged and this varicosity gives purplish blue colour to the affected part. Later on these parts change to ulcers which are indurated, hard, suppurated or malignant. Induration and infiltration of the various parts due to ulcers. These ulcers ooze acrid discharge. Tearing type of headache, congestion and confusion. Local or general lymphadenopathy.

Patient is very anxious and sad. Palpitation. She is confused and can't clear her ideas about anything. She wants to be alone. Great aversion to company. Does not like to talk to anybody.

MODALITIES :

< Night, touch, bleeding.

> When sitting alone.

4.4.5 THUJA

Cauliflower-like overgrowth at the cervical os which bleeds easily on touch. Congestion of the parts with chronic discharge from the genital tract, which are thick greenish and profuse. Severe pain in the left ovarian and left inguinal region.

CARCINOMA CERVIX

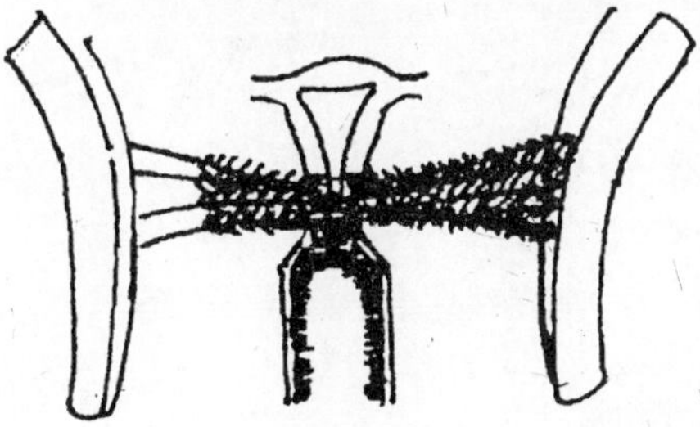

Stage. III : Ca. extended on to the pelvic wall.

Exocervical carcinoma has a tendency to spread superficially over the vaginal surface of cervix, to right and left fornices. Therefore there are chances of invasion or infiltration of vaginal wall. Endocervical carcinoma grows into the cervix to infiltrate it. It forms barrel shaped cervix which is hard in nature and occasionally associated with small overgrowths in the form of tumours. These overgrowths further spread into uterine region.

Menses are scanty and retarded. Loss of appetite with bitter and rancid eructations. Chronic dyspepsia due to malignancy. There is a vascular, papillary growth or malignant ulcer is visible in the cervical os. Ill- effects of suppressed gonorrhoea or other sexually transmitted diseases. There is tearing and cutting pain in urethra with sensation as if urine is constantly flowing. Frequent desire to pass urine. Dysuria. Thick yellowish, glitty, bloody discharges from urethra. Skin is prone to get warts, condylomata and other types of overgrowth. Skin is dry with herpetic eruptions. Sometimes sweat has sweetish odour.

Patient has desire to remain alone. Doesn't want company or to mix with people. Very quarrelsome and irritable. Thuja lady has a kind of strange, fixed notions or ideas in her mind, like she is pregnant or something live is moving in abdomen or somebody is following her. Mental ailments due to hormonal imbalance.

MODALITIES :

< From touch, heat of bed, at night times, cold and damp weather.

> Open air.

****

CHAPTER 5

DISEASES OF UTERUS

TOPIC 1

ENDOMETRITIS

5.1.1 PULSATILLA

This remedy is well-known for suppression of the menses. This suppression is due to getting feet wet. Amenorrhoea may give rise to infection. The hormonal imbalance may suppress the menses. The vessels of the uterus show the picture of acute inflammation with various signs and symptoms of endometritis. Abdomen is painful, distended with loud rumbling. Sensation as if pressed by a stone. Severe intestinal colic. Shooting type of pain in the sacrum which travel upwards in between the shoulders.

The mucous membranes especially of uterus are affected with severe inflammation. This results in leucorrhoea which is acrid, burning and creamy. Severe backache and sense of tiredness. Wandering, stitching pains in the head which extends to face. Dry mouth without thirst. Cutting pains in abdomen with urging for stool. Haemorrhoids with constipation. Catarrhal condition of the chest. Asthmatic or oppressed breathing. Sense of tightness in the chest. The pains in the extremities are wandering in nature. Drawing and tearing pains which are worse by warmth. This remedy is indicated for threatened abortion. The endometritis which is secondary to abortion is best treated by this remedy.

Mental symptoms are worse in warm room and better in open air. She is very afraid to meet males and thus dislikes to get married. Patient is very religious, constantly dwells upon religious things. She is in general mild, gentle, sad and timid with weeping tendency.

MODALITIES :

< Warmth in general, in warm room, after eating rich fatty food.

> Open air, cold application, cold drinks etc.

5.1.2 CARBO ANIMALIS

Induration of the endometrium of the uterus. This inflammation gives pressing pains in the loins. Inflammation of the complete genital tract. This causes burning of labia, vagina and uterine region. Increase of secretions due to inflammatory conditions of endometrium. Yellowish staining on the clothes due to leucorrhoea. Ascending type of infection with rise of temperature. There is abdominal discomfort with burning and griping pain in abdomen. Weak digestion with flatulency. The mucous membrane of the uterus becomes oedematous, thick and hyperaemic.

Patient has scrofulous constitution and is inclined to menopause. She had suffered from many debilitating diseases. All the secretions are offensive. Mostly causes local congestion without fever. There is headache with confused hearing. Weak, empty feeling in the stomach. Various lymph nodes, glands are indurated and swollen. Tearing pains running transversely across the pubis and then goes up to anus.

Mentally the patient is cheerful and has despondency. She prefers to be alone. Does not want to talk or to be questioned. She is very anxious especially at night.

MODALITIES :

< All the symptoms are aggravated due to loss of animal fluid and at night.

> When alone.

5.1.3 AURUM MUR. NAT.

This remedy is useful in chronic inflammatory conditions of the mucous membrane of uterus. Inflammation of the endocervix moves and settles in fundus of uterus. Flexions from condensation of uterine tissue or from softening of the stroma of the body of uterus. Habitual abortions or miscarriages constantly bring about induration in some part of the uterus preventing natural expansions. Ulcers on wall of the uterus when exposed to various infections cause endometritis. There is swelling and induration of the cervical canal. Leucorrhoea with spasmodic contractions of vagina. Ovaries are indurated. Subinvolution, swelled uterus fills up the whole of pelvis.

She complains of high blood pressure due to disturbed functions of nervous mechanism. There is arteriosclerosis. Syphilitic ataxia.

5.1.4 BOVISTA

Uterine engorgement from relaxation of entire capillary system. She has haemorrhagic diathesis and bleeds profusely. Menorrhagia. Also there is metrorrhagia. Menses too early and profuse. Bleeding especially at night times. Condition usually seen in nonpuerperal cases. Due to profuse bleeding there is malaise and sometimes feeling of chill is prominent present. Flow of blood between menses from least exertion and at night and also in early morning is chief guiding symptom of Bovista.

Due to inflammatory condition of the uterus, there is soreness of pubis during menses. Abdominal colic or haematuria. Colicky pain relieved by eating. She has to bend double to get rid of abdominal pain. Sensation as if head were enlarging especially the occiput. Dull, bruised pain in the brain. Cheeks and lips feel swollen. Sensation as if lump of ice in abdomen.

Patient has strange feeling of enlargement. She is awkward and drops everything from hand. Very sensitive.

MODALITIES :

< Tight clothing around waist

> Rest

5.1.5 BELLADONNA

Acute inflammatory condition of the endometrium. Recent prolapse especially after parturition makes the uterine walls indurated. Cervical mucous membrane is very congested and red. Bearing down pains as if everything would come out of the vulva. There is dryness and heat of vagina. Cutting pain from hip to hip. Menses and lochia are very offensive and hot. She complains of severe backache as if the back would break.There is inflammation of ovaries, fallopian tubes, uterus with high degree of fever.

Dry, hot skin which is very sensitive, with burning. High feverish state with comparative absence of toxaemia. Burning, steaming heat but feet are icy cold. No thirst during fever.

Patient is restless and has a tendency to cry out. She has visual hallucinations. Loss of conciousness and disinclined to talk. Vertigo with tendency to fall on left side or backwards.

MODALITIES :

< Movement, pressure.

> Rest in lying with head elevated.

5.1.6 CONVALLARIA MAJALIS

Great soreness in uterine region due to inflammation of the uterus. This is due to prolapse of uterus or criminal abortion which sets the secondary infection. There is severe backache and also pain in the lumbar region which extends to lower limbs. Sore, aching pains in lower part of abdomen with feeling as if uterus has descended and pressed upon rectum. It causes hard aching pain in rectum and anus. During menstruation, pains in sacro-iliac joint running down the legs. With endometritis, there is distressing itching at vaginal orifice and urethral meatus.

This is popularly a heart remedy; when selected upon totality of symptoms, increases energy of heart. Patient presents with rawness and soreness of lips, nose. Sometimes epistaxis. There is pulmonary congestion with orthopnoea. Dyspnoea while walking.

MODALITIES :

< In warm room.

> Open air.

Other important remedies for endometritis are

1) FERRUM PHOS.
2) SILICEA
3) HELONIAS
4) BORAX
5) HEPAR SULPH.
6) MERC SOL.
7) ARSENICUM ALBUM
8) RHUS TOX.

============

TOPIC 2

PROLAPSE OF UTERUS

5.2.1 COLLINSONIA

During pregnancy, Collinsonia patient suffers from obstinate constipation. There is feeling of obstruction. To overcome this feeling and pass the faeces patient has to strain much. This straining results in prolapse of uterus. During labour there is incompetency of the os. Therefore she has to strain to deliver. This also contributes to the prolapse of uterus. Abnormal tonicity of the muscular fibres of uterus is observed. Pruritus in pregnancy is marked and or guiding symptom of this remedy. Due to overstraining during labour, she complains of bleeding piles with intense stitching pains.

Patient complains of pruritus vulvae. There is feeling of swelling of clitoris and labial muscles. Bowels are constipated, evacuates in the form of lumps but to complete the act she has to strain much. There are pains in anus and in hypogastrium after stool. Bleeding and stitching pains after stool due to engorged piles. Many a time constipation alternates with diarrhoea which is bloody and contains mucus. There are intense spasmodic pains in the rectal region and in descending colon. Dull, frontal headache if the bleeding from haemorrhoids is suppressed.

Patient is emotional and excited very easily due to trifling reasons. Confused and irritable.

MODALITIES :

< Mental emotions and mental distress, cold in general.

> Rest in bed, heat in general.

5.2.2 PODOPHYLLUM

Prolapse of uterus due to pouring diarrhoea and also due to overlifting and after parturition. Patient has long-standing diarrhoea which aggravates early in the morning. Diarrhoea of the Podophyllum is very characteristic and can be remembered with " Five Ps", they are profuse, painless, putrid, polychromatic and prolapsing. Prolapse of uterus due to chronic dehydration and loss of muscular elasticity. Labour is very much difficult and she has to strain for that, therefore the Podophyllum lady complains of prolapse of uterus after parturition. There is laxity and atony of pelvic supports. There is bearing down sensation and the cervix lies at the level of external os. This is "second degree" of uterine prolapse.

Numb, aching pains in the right ovarian region and also in the right hypochondriac region. There is distension of the abdomen. Gaseous distension of abdomen and patient can lie comfortably on abdomen as abdominal colic is ameliorated by pressure. Tongue is flabby and moist. With prolapse of uterus, there is leucorrhoea which is thick, transparent and in the mucous form. Nocturnal urination is marked due to prolapse of uterus.

Patient has great loquacity during diarrhoea and prolapse of uterus. Delirious. She is very depressed.

MODALITIES :

< Early in the morning, hot weather.

> Lying on abdomen.

5.2.3 SEPIA

Pelvic organs are relaxed and there is bearing down sensation as if the uterus would escape through vaginal opening. She must cross her limbs to prevent protruding or apply some pressure on genitalia. There is atonic relaxation of the supports of uterus especially broad ligament of the uterus and stretching and tearing of pelvic fascia lead to widening of vaginal canal or introitus. Damage of the pelvic supports at childbirth is one of the factors responsible for the prolapse. Bearing down sensation is worse when sitting, while standing, on walking. With pelvic protrusion, there is leucorrhoea which is yellowish green in colour, causes intense itching of vulval region with redness, swelling and eruptions. Complete procidentia, that is, the uterus lies outside the vagina.

With the uterus, bladder also comes out which causes increased frequency of micturition. The patient narrates that she has to push the uterus up manually to complete the act of micturition. Patient has vertigo with sensation as if something rolling around head. Dry cough, usually more in the evening and after lying down at night. There is intense pain in stomach with nausea and bitter taste in the mouth after vomiting. Menses are suppressed, too late and scanty. They are irregular also. Patient has urging to urinate from pressure of uterus on the bladder. Loud rumbling in the abdomen. The lady presents with pale face which is yellowish red and flushed.

Patient is excessively nervous, depressed and absent-minded. She is very irritable, fearful and easily offended. Indifferent to whom she loved best. Wants company, afraid to be alone. Misery, weeps frequently while narrating her complaints.

MODALITIES :

- < In afternoon, in evening, after having food, while sitting and walking.
- > In open air, by sitting legs crossed.

5.2.4 LILIUM TIGRINUM

Uterine symptoms usually follow pregnancy and labour. There is bearing down sensation of the uterus. Heavy weight and pressure in the uterine region. Early bearing down sensation during parturition when the foetal head still lies at the level of cervix with improper cervical dilatation. The cervix descends with the uterine body from their normal position into the vagina and afterwards the cervix protrudes outside the vaginal introitus. This many a time is associated with cystocele, rectocele and relaxed perineum. Heaviness, dragging sensation principally in hypogastric region. Patient gets feeling as if she needs something to support genital organs and prevent their prolapse. Fundus of uterus lowers down and tilts against bladder, automatically the cervical os presses upon the rectum. Bearing down pains in the uterine region.

Impairment of vitality in the ladies who have uterine neuralgia. Heaviness of the head with staggering, faint feeling, oppressed breathing with nervous trembling. Abdomen is distended and there is sensation as if diarrhoea will set in at any moment. There is pressure of cervical os on rectum with almost constant desire for defecation. There are smarting, burning pains in the anus with frequent urination during daytime.

Patient has depression of the spirits which results in weeping. She is very apprehensive and timid. She has the feeling she has to complete many things so she has to hurry, work urgently. Also there is fear that she is unable to complete it. She has inclination to think of obscene things as there is uterine irritation.

MODALITIES :

< In the evening, at night, by losing self-control.

> During daytime, from fresh air, by keeping herself busy in work, warmth in general, warm room, warm drinks and warm clothings.

5.2.5 AGARICUS MUSCARIUS

Genital prolapse results from failure of support to pelvic organs, precipitated by raised abdominal pressure and cessation of menses. There is descent of uterus along with the rectal wall with middl part of the posterior vaginal wall. After prolonged time this rectal wall protrudes outside the vaginal orifice. There is history of incomplete perineal tear. Cystocele also is very common in Agaricus. Troubles generally start after cessation of the menses with intolerable bearing down pains. There are cramps in the uterine region as if she is going to deliver a baby. There is intense itching with irritation of the parts. Patient narrates the complaints as awful bearing down pains which are beyond her capacity to tolerate. There is itching and irritation of the external genitalia.

PROLAPSE OF UTERUS

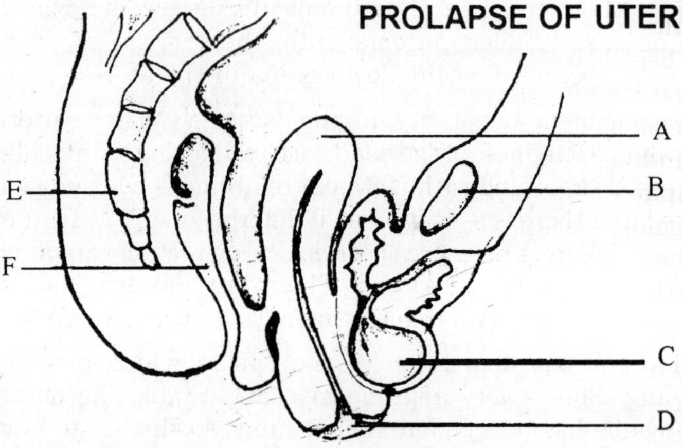

A. Uterus B. Symphysis pubis C. Bladder
D. Prolapse cervix E. Coccyx F. Rectum

With prolapse of uterus, patient also complains of stiffness in nape of neck and a funny sensation of stiffness between the shoulders. Pains radiate up and down the lumbar region. Tremors of the hand. Twitching of different group of muscles. Repeated sneezing and loud coughing. Worse forenoon. Expectoration of ball of mucus. Patient is hungry but no desire for food. Sour eructation with stitching type of pain in the liver region. Pimples are converted to vesicles containing yellow serum. Shortsighted lady. Motion of letters while reading.

Mentally the patient is delirious with always raving. Exhausted; wants to leave the bed. Patient is indifferent, ill humoured and very stubborn. Self-willed and does not like to answer questions.

MODALITIES :

< In winter, before a thunderstorm, open air, after taking food, after coitus.

> Walking gently.

5.2.6 ALOE SOCOTRINE

Patient is very exhausted and has sedentary habits. It causes haemorrhoids and also rectocele which ultimately results in the prolapse of uterus due to pressure on it. Patient has bearing down pains in rectum with incontinence of urine. Sense of heaviness in uterus across groins and loins. Piles and headache are alternating with lumbago. Pains in back are extending down the legs. Feels as if there is a plug between symphysis pubis and os coccygis. Uterus has heaviness and dragging down pains when prolapse occurs especially in women of menopause. Mostly associated with morning diarrhoea.

Patient is having sense of insecurity in the rectum. Sedentary habit also leads to bland purplish piles usually in grape-like bunches. Headache with heaviness in eyes and has to close them. Headache alternates with lumbago. Great flatulence. Dyspnoea with winter cough. Bitter taste in mouth. Epistaxis.

Patient is very irritable and excited on any matter. Suitable to retired persons who are having sedentary life. Patient is at menopause but dissatisfied about everything in her life and in other persons also.

MODALITIES :

< After eating and drinking, hot weather, in morning.

> Cold application, cold open air.

5.2.7 CALCAREA CARB

As the Calcarea carb patient is fat, fair, flabby, there are two factors thus appear operating in the mechanism of prolapse of uterus. First is the failure of the pelvic supports, which pushes the uterus down. Secondly the increased abdominal pressure bears down the anterior vaginal wall followed by cervix and then the posterior vaginal wall. The cystocele is very common in Calcarea carb patient as the bladder descends along with the uterus. The Calcarea patient has obstinate constipation, the stools are hard and knotty and they are to be removed mechanically. To overcome this trouble, patient goes on straining and becomes victim of prolapse of uterus. There is frequency of micturition during daytime when the patient is in standing position. When patient lies down frequency decreases. This frequency of micturition is due to difficulty in emptying the bladder. The stress incontinence can also be seen. Leucorrhoea may be due to associated cervicitis with mild degree of vaginitis. Metrorrhoea may occur due to decubitus ulcers.

Menses are too early, last too long and are too profuse. Milky discharges from vagina. Piles protrude out which causes pains during stools. There is feeling of heaviness in lower part of rectum. Abdomen is hard and very much distended. On physical exertion the lower part of abdomen is distended with spasmodic pains. Patient is very hungry in the morning. There is great thirst with frequent eructations. Pit of stomach is swollen and looks like inverted saucer. Pressure in the stomach as if a lump in it. This causes pressure on uterus. Tickling cough with sensation of a feather in throat. Oppressed breathing with expectoration of mucus having sweetish taste.

Patient is sleepless due to great anxiety with palpitation of the heart. Does not like to start work and has tendency to avoid it. She is frightful and apprehensive.

MODALITIES :

< In morning, from cold in general, after eating, from exertion.

> Warmth in general, dry climate, lying down.

Other important remedies for prolapse or uterus are

1. PLATINA
2. PULSATILLA
3. RHUS TOX.
4. PALADIUM
5. LACHESIS
6. LILIUM TIG.

============

TOPIC 3
TUMOUR OF UTERUS

5.3.1 SILICEA

As the remedy falls in sycotic group, it has tendency to overgrowth. The actual reason for overgrowth is not known. But tumours of uterus arise from endometrial hyperplasia. Sometimes the tumour is of muscle tissues in origin. These muscle tissues are matured muscle fibres. Intramural growth is commonly seen in majority of cases. This remedy acts powerfully upon vegetative form of the disease and affects especially organic substances of the body, more often the mucous surface. If it is a benign growth of uterus such as fibroid or fibromyoma then the growth is insidious with menorrhagia. Menses are too early, too profuse and acrid. Due to increased proliferation of tissues and the congestion of the tissues, there is leucorrhoea which is corrosive in nature, milky and mucopurulent. Due to the heaviness of uterus, there is sense of bearing down or pressing down of the uterus in the vaginal vault. Itching of the genitals and parts are tender to touch.

Increased frequency of micturition with distress from improper functioning of the sphincter of urethra. Nipples are ulcerated and are very tender. Vertigo associated with congestion of head. Patient complains of headache which start on nape of neck, spreads over head and settles over eyebrows. Itching pustules on scalp and neck better from wrapping up warmly. Ravenous hunger. She is disgusted with meat and warm food. Cramp in calf muscles and sciatica.

Mentally patient is very timid and unstable. She feels it difficult to concentrate her mind. She is confused and restless.

Worried about the future. Yielding disposition but nervous. She is very sensitive to external impressions.

MODALITIES :

< In morning, after washing the parts, during flow, uncovering, rest in bed.

> Warmth in general, damp wet weather.

5.3.2 THUJA OCCIDENTALIS –

The benign tumours of the uterus, subserous or intramural have got tendency to go malignant. These tumours lie underneath the peritoneum. Sometimes they are sessile or sometimes pedunculated. They are adherent to surrounding

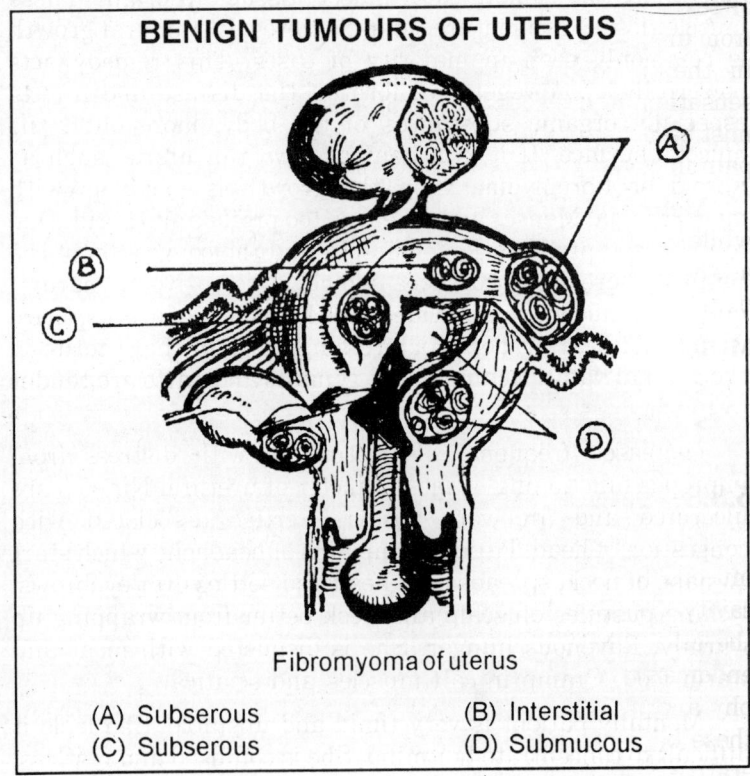

BENIGN TUMOURS OF UTERUS

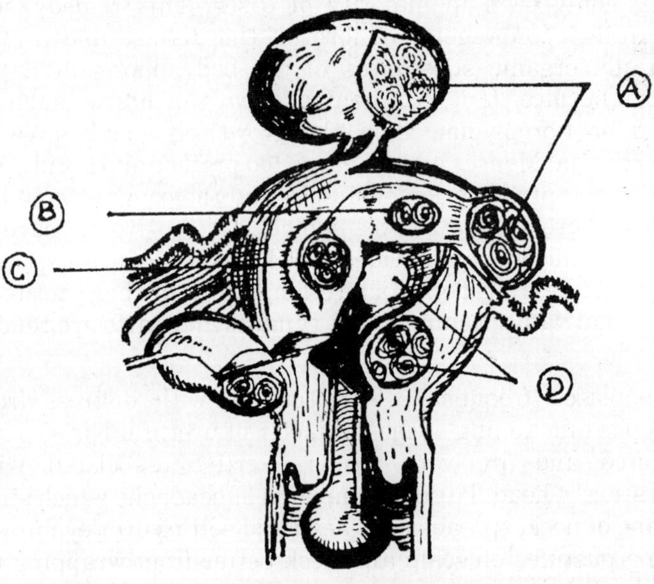

Fibromyoma of uterus

(A) Subserous (B) Interstitial
(C) Subserous (D) Submucous

structures. Spherical in shape and firm in consistancy. Due to the excessive blood supply to fibroids there is congestion of uterine wall. This causes profuse bleeding with stitching pains in abdomen. Leucorrhoea which is yellowish green in nature. When secondary infection sets in, there is inflammation of vagina hence vagina, becomes very much sensitive especially during the act of coitus. Polypoid growth of the uterus turns into cauliflower-like growth which bleeds easily. Severe backache while walking. Menses are too short and too early preceded by profuse perspiration.

Due to the pressure of fibroid on urinary bladder there is frequent urging to urinate. This increase in frequency of micturition, usually at night times, is characteristic of Thuja lady. Boring pain in the region of bladder. She gives history of sexually transmitted disease with thick, gleety discharge from urethra with burning. Aphthous ulcer in the mouth. Pain in the left frontal region or right temporal region with sensation as if a nail were driven in. Dimness of vision, as if mist before eyes. Jerking of the upper extremities and crampy pain in lower extremities. She has tendency to develop warts.

Mentally she is absent-minded and makes many mistakes while talking. Many a time she omits the words while writing as she cannot think fast. She has to talk very slowly, still she uses wrong words while talking.

MODALITIES :

< In the morning, heat of bed.

> Open air, warmth in general, by movement.

5.3.3 PHOSPHORUS

Growth of fibroid, submucous type growths under the mucous membrane of uterus which project inside the uterine cavity. It is usually single in number and sessile. Due to this, the cavity of the uterus enlarges. There may be associated endometrial hyperplasia with endometritis. There is hypertrophy and inflammation of blood vessels of the uterus. When these benign tumours change to malignancy, hyaline degenerative changes can be observed. These changes can be seen after menopause. Due to overgrowth of fibroids, there is prolapse of uterus with weak, sinking feeling in the abdomen. Pains in the uterus have tendency to run upwards. Due to inflammatory conditions there are stitching and throbbing pains in uterus or vagina. Menses are profuse and too late. Leucorrhoea is acrid in nature, presents instead of menses. Cancer of the uterus can be well treated by this remedy if the symptoms match correctly.

Tall, slender ladies and those who are narrow chested are prone to get the diseases of the uterus. She has ravenous hunger specially at night but she complains of sour eructations after eating. Desire for cold water, but vomits it out as soon as it gets warm in stomach. But in general all symptoms are relieved by warmth and aggravated by cold. There is intense burning everywhere. Periodical headache. Congestive or neuralgic type, associated with vertigo. Dandruff and alopecia. Swelling of both the eyelids, sensation as if everything is covered with a mist. Blue rings around the eyes. Fan-like motion of alae nasi. Epistaxis, vicarious menstruation. Nose is full of mucus with little haemorrhages. All-gone sensation in head, chest and abdomen. Heat is felt between scapulae. Stitching and burning pains in joints. Weak and numb feeling in upper extremities with rheumatism of joints.

Mentally the patient is having debility of mind and weak memory with weeping tendency. But she becomes irritable; sees something creeping out from every corner of room. Fearful and anxious. Apprehension; indifferent to persons in good relation. Delirium, sadness, melancholia with hysteria. She suddenly behaves like a fool and becomes violent. Brain-fag, fear of death.

MODALITIES :

< Twilight, during thunderstorm, lying on left side, pressure, any work, warm food or drink.

> Lying on right side, cold food, cold drink, cold open air, darkness, sleep.

5.3.4 GRAPHITES

Graphites lady is psoric in nature. Engorgement of the veins, lymphatic vessels and hardness of the cervical canal. Whole thickness of the cervical canal is stiffened. Normal stratification of epithelium is lost. The endometrium lining of the uterus is swollen and is covered with leucocytic and round cell infiltration. They show large hyperchromatic, irregular nuclei and abnormal mitosis. Big tumours, size of an orange, can be palpable in right and left fornices. Pain in the uterus with bearing down sensation. Vagina is cold. Cicatric tissue easily cracks and bleeds. Pain in the hypogastric region like an electric shock. Leucorrhoea instead of menses. Discharge is offensive, white and excoriating.

Graphites lady is anaemic or chlorotic. She suffers from various skin eruptions like erysipelas, eczema or herpes. All eruptions ooze a sticky exudation. Every little injury has tendency to suppurate. Cracked labial commissures, nipples and other places. The lady is very much sensitive to pains and has ophthalmia, blephritis. May present with oedema of legs and thick, crippled, brittle nails. Pain in sternal region with sense of constriction in chest. Nocturnal attacks of spasmodic asthma. Distension and hardness in abdomen so she loosens the clothing. Nausea, and croaking in abdomen. Flatulence. Chronic diarrhoea or lienteria, which is very offensive. Haemorrhoids and prolapse of rectum with fissure in anus.

Patient is very irritable and gets easily excited for minor things. She has no desire to work or even to think. She is very sad and apprehensive. Hurried to start any work but indecisive and despondent. In the morning sluggishness is well observed. She is aggravated from hearing music, it causes her to weep and she gets depressed.

MODALITIES :

< During and after menses, warmth in general, night, eating and music.

> Open air, darkness, covering.

5.3.5 THLASPI BURSA PASTORIS CAPSELLA

This remedy is used in the diseases of uterus like carcinoma of uterus, fibroids of uterus with profuse haemorrhage, usually frequent. Haemorrhage in the form of clots. Brownish coloured. Pain in the uterine region due to overgrowth. Intense backache and general bruised soreness. Lady complains of various uterine diseases and suppression of the same by the use of medicines of other schools. Metrorrhagia, too frequent, copious haemorrhages with violent uterine colic. Every alternate period is very painful and she bleeds profusely. Leucorrhoea before and after menstruation. It is bloody, dark and offensive. There is frequent desire for urination. Urethritis, usually associated with the uterine problems.

Patient has aching between the scapulae or whole back and in general she has bruised soreness everywhere. She has frequent, profuse haemorrhages from every natural orifice. Passive bleeding from nose, epistaxis. White tongue; cracks in mouth and lips. Face is puffy and neuralgic, sharp pain over right eye, vertigo. Renal colic with albuminuria or haematuria. Urethra is very much inflamed so dysuria and spasmodic retention of urine. She has frequent desire for urination. Urine shows brick-dust sediment.

Patient is very worried and anxious about her complaints. There is sulggishness of thoughts. General dizziness due to haemorrhage.

5.3.6 SABINA

Sabina is covered under sycotic miasm, thus lady complains of overgrowths in the uterine region. In the carcinoma of uterus, she has cauliflower-like growth which usually occurs by direct spread. Exocervical carcinoma tends to spread superficially on the endometrial surface. It may also take place by lymphatic spread. It occurs by permeation or embolism. The obturator lymph nodes get affected first followed by external iliac and internal iliac lymph nodes. Menstrual cycles are disturbed. Menses are profuse and blood is bright red in colour. Uterine pains extend up to thighs. Discharges of blood between periods with sexual excitement. Pains from sacrum to pubis is characteristic symptom of Sabina lady. Uterine haemorrhage is partly clotted and aggravated by least motion.

After the haemorrhage, there are very violent pulsations with sense of fullness in the veins in peripheral organs. Haemorrhoids are bleeding profusely with bright red blood. Constipation and haematuria. Bitter taste with burning in the pit of stomach. Colic with tympanic distension and bearing down pains. Gouts are seen everywhere. Congestion of head and face. Toothache while chewing food. Bursting type of headache with pulsations, sudden onset and insidious cessation. Vertigo associated with suppressed menses. Burning and throbbing pains in the kidney region.

MODALITIES :

< Least motion, warmth in general, hot air, hot climate.

> Cold fresh air, rest.

5.3.7 LACHESIS

Lachesis has got affinity for malignant growths. Mainly she has tendency to malignancy especially during the climaxis. The growth alters the hormonal levels and before menses she may have fainting spells. Menses are of short duration and flow is scanty. Flow is dark, non-clotted blood. Flow is watery. Regularity of menses is well maintained in this patient. This regular flow of menses relieves many of her complaints. Metrorrhagia is marked.

She is very hot and cannot bear heat in any form. She has flushes of heat all over the body. Her built is thin and emaciated with bluish circles around the eyes. All her complaints are aggravated during and after sleep. The abdomen or pelvic region is very sensitive to touch and she cannot bear even the touch of clothing around her waist. Cramps in abdomen. Great palpitation with tendency to bleed from every orifice.

Mental sphere of Lachesis lady is very similar to mental disturbances of female patients. She is very jealous and suspicious. Marked irritability and talkative nature with religious insanity. Melancholy with weak memory. Dreams of snakes.

MODALITIES :

< During and after sleep, tight clothes around waist, lying on left side, warmth in general.

> Open air, discharges.

Other important remedies for tumour of uterus are as follows :-

1. IODINE
2. KREOSOTUM
3. CALENDULA
4. LYCOPODIUM
5. IGNATIA

============

TOPIC 4

DYSFUNCTIONAL UTERINE BLEEDING (DUB)

5.4.1 TRILLIUM PENDULUM

This is a general antihaemorrhagic remedy. Active haemorrhage from the uterus, of dark coloured blood, sometimes in the form of clots and sometimes thick, sticky in nature. Oozes continuously from the uterus for several days. There is prolonged bleeding often preceded by amenorrhoea for a month or two. Painless bleeding. This is commonly seen in premenopause and in adolescence. Usually the cause is menstrual endocrine dysfunction due to failure of LH. This is also suited for women who invariably bleed after parturition or miscarriage. Gushing of bright red blood from the uterine cavity at every little movement which makes the patient pale as from anaemia. Menses usually after overexertion, long journey, travelling etc. There is sense of giddiness after bleeding. Abnormal uterine growth such as fibroids, polyps etc. stimulate bleeding. There is great bearing down sensation with copious leucorrhoea.

Trillium lady shows profuse blood loss from each and every orifice. Due to this blood loss, she may have attack of dyspnoea with chest pain. Lady is initially plethoric but due to the haemorrhages, she becomes wasted and cachectic. Profuse blood loss at the menopausal age is well treated by this remedy. Blood loss is in the form of chronic excessive menstrual bleeding. Passive intermenstrual bleeding, i.e. menorrhagia. She has tendency to uterine outgrowths. After the haemorrhage, she has dizziness or she may faint if the blood loss is excessive. She has varicosity with sense of tightness in the veins of lower parts.

5.4.2 SECALE COR.

Burning pain in the uterus, with irregular menstrual bleeding. Continuous oozing of watery blood from the uterus till next period. Haemorrhage with strong and spasmodic contraction of the uterus. Flow of blood is preceded by strong bearing down pains. Haemorrhage in Secale cor. is usually due to atony of uterus, after parturition or miscarriage. Bleeding is more after movements. Bleeding is passive, of dark colour and is continuous in nature. Non-coagulable, offensive in nature. She has tendency to threatened abortion in or about third month. Labour is prolonged. Uterus is relaxed. No expulsive movements therefore goes on bleeding for longer time. Dark, offensive lochia. Putrid discharges; coldness of the parts, profuse perspiration. Pains with numbness and tingling sensation in the extremities. Metrorrhagia with the sensation of a string or a clot.

Secale cor. patient is always very hot and she may have history of exposure to very hot climate for long duration. She feels intolerable heat everywhere in the body. Vessels and the muscles are very relaxed and atonic, this leads to flooding of the parts. She has dried up look. Along with the menorrhagia she has great depression of mind. She has coldness of the body. Then also she does not like to be covered. Increased thirst and hunger. Dyspnoea and palpitation. General anaemic condition with coldness, numbness and tired feeling. Eats much but cannot gain weight. Instead of weight gain she becomes cachetic. Melancholic lady.

MODALITIES :

< Heat in general, covering.

> Cold in general, rubbing, open air and uncovering.

5.4.3 LYCOPODIUM

Irregular bleeding during climaxis. Chronic catarrhal condition of the uterus. Chronic inflammation of the endometrium due to infections. Prolonged uterine bleeding due to myohyperplasia and glandular hyperplasia in the uterus. Uterus becomes uniformly enlarged due to this myohyperplasia and the endometrium becomes markedly grown, thick and vascular in nature. Obstinate leucorrhoea is associated with this haemorrhage. Menses are too late and last too long. She bleeds profusely. Vagina is dry, enlargement of the right ovary causes severe pain in right fornix. There is varicosity of the veins of pudenda associated with acrid and burning leucorrhoea. Cutting pains across the abdomen from right to left with rumbling in upper part which descends to lower parts. Bleeding is profuse and protracted flow, partly black, clotted and partly bright red. Increased blood flow from vagina during every passage of hard and soft stool.

Lycopodium lady has got multiple congestive spots everywhere in the body with hampered circulation. Patient is very chilly due to lack of vital heat. She has great aversion for cold things. Frequent dyspnoea with palpitation and violent cough in night. Sudden onset and cessation of the pains. Dyspepsia with great flatulence. Drowsy feeling during whole day. Dropsical condition everywhere.

Confusion with weak memory. Obstinate lady with melancholy. Oversensitive and irritable. Sadness and great apprehension. Feels that her brain is weakening.

MODALITIES :

< 4-8 p.m., cold in general.

> Early in morning, heat in general, warm air, movements.

5.4.4 HAMAMELIS VIRGINICA

This is a suitable remedy for venous congestion and haemorrhages. Ovarian congestion and neuralgia. Inflammation of the endometrium of the uterus. It becomes thick, vascular and polypoid. There are no secretory changes in the endometrium. This type of character correlates with this remedy, therefore the haemorrhage continues for a longer time. Bleeding is steady and slow. Blood is dark, black coloured without any pains in the uterus. Blood flow is usually seen in the daytime and almost absent during the night. There is hammering type of headache associated with bleeding. There are bearing down pains in back during haemorrhage. Lady is prone to bleed in between the periods. Intense itching of the vulva.

Vicarious menstruation, haematemesis and haemorrhoids are the other features of venous congestion of Hamamelis lady. She has throbbing or pulsating pains in the affected parts. There is marked distruction of the epithelium of the uterus and it is accompanied with great soreness and pains. Severe backache and weak feeling of extremities. Sense of constriction around the chest and tickling sensation in throat excites the cough.

MODALITIES :

< Exertion, warmth in general, motion, moist air.

> Open air.

5.4.5 IPECACUANHA

Uterine haemorrhage is profuse, bright red and gushing, with constant nausea. This nausea is not at all relieved by vomiting. Nausea proceeds from the stomach. The discharge of bright red blood from the uterus is increased with every effort to vomit. Violent pressure on the uterus by the abdominal viscera. Irregular shedding of the endometrial lining occurs due to retrogression of corpus luteum. Woman bleeds irregularly following menstruation. Faintness after profuse bleeding. Bleeding is worse when getting out of the bed. Bleeding from the uterus soaks the bed-cloths. Pain in the navel, passing through the uterus.

Skin is very much pale and relaxed. Clean tongue, ptyalism and thirstlessness though she has constant nausea and vomiting. Blueness around the eyes. Dyspnoea in a chilly lady, with catching of the breath and uterine colic. Eyes are half open.

Spasms everywhere in the body. Catches cold very easily.

She is oversensitive to external impressions. Very short tempered and loses control easily. She has desire for many things but does not know what.

MODALITIES :

< Lying down, movement in winter season (periodical), cold.

> By rest.

5.4.6 BELLADONNA

Profuse discharge of bright red blood from the uterus, which feels hot to the thighs. During labour the uterus shows hour glass contraction and placenta is retained so uterus bleeds profusely. The blood is always bright red in colour. Uterus is congested and she has uterine colic. Very strong bearing down pains. Uterus is relaxed, so veins are dilated and bleed copiously. There is great soreness in the uterus with sensation of heaviness. She has to sit and cannot lie down due to the sense of heaviness. Parts are very much sensitive.

Belladonna lady is extremely sensitive and is plethoric. She has congestion in every part of the body. Right side of the uterus, right tube and right ovary are more affected. She has irritation and soreness in the portio vaginalis. All the discharges and blood feel very hot.

Hot, distended and painful abdomen, especially on the right side. Urine is retained after labour and she feels that there is warmth in her bladder. Easy and violent palpitation and throbbing pulse everywhere in the body. Lumbago and the pains spread to the hips and thighs. Restless lady with irresistible cries due to intense pains. Tightness with sense of constriction in the abdomen. Throbbing type of headache with vertigo.

Mind is in a state of violence and she becomes maniac and offends everybody. She disturbs everybody either by speech or by action.

She is hypersensitive to every stimuli. Unconciousness.

MODALITIES :

< Any external stimuli, touch, jar.

> When she sits in semi-erect position.

5.4.7 APOCYNUM CANNABINUM

This remedy induces or stimulates the secretions of mucous and serous membranes producing oedema and dropsy. She has metrorrhagia with nausea, fainting and vital depression. Haemorrhage at the time of menopause. Blood expelled in large clots. Atrophied endometrium causes irregular breathing in old patients. The endometrium is very thin and has poor proliferation with few atrophic glands. The ovarian function of secretion of hormone is lost. Efforts at vomiting cause profuse bleeding. Great prostration and trembling of the whole body. For one or two days, the bleeding seems to reduce in quantity; but it then again increases. She complains of fainting when raising the head from pillow. Great exhaustion of the vital powers. Great irritability of the stomach causes vomiting. Palpitation when she attempts to move, with profuse haemorrhage.

There is feeling she is free from all the complaints at times but then she again suffers from involuntary and profuse diarrhoea. Retention of urine with great urging and the quantity of urine is very scanty. Sometimes she has involuntary urination. Violent palpitation, and she faints when head is raised. Pulse is very weak and thready.

Lady is very low spirited and mannerless. Behaves like a wild entity. Restless and sleepless.

MODALITIES :

< Uncovering the parts, cold application, cold air.

Other useful remedies for dysfunctional uterine bleeding are

1) THLASPI BURSA PASTORIS
2) CALCAREA CARBONICA
3) PHOSPHORUS
4) NITRIC ACID
5) HELONIAS

****

CHAPTER 6

DISEASES OF BREAST

TOPIC 1
TUMOUR OF BREAST

6.1.1 CONIUM MACULATUM

Mammary glands are hard and sore. A typical carcinoma of the breast, that is, scirrhous adenocarcinoma, which begins in the ducts and ends in the parenchyma. As the stage advances the Cooper's ligament shortens and thus it produces the notch. Sometimes the condition is associated with the inflammation of the breast tissue. The region is hard and nodular, tender to touch. Burning and stinging pains in the breast. The skin over the tumour is adherent. Occasionally there is discharge of pus from the nipple. The lesion is hard, almost cartilaginous. The edges are distinct, serrated and irregular; associated with productive fibrosis.

Patient is greatly debilitated and there is tiredness of the mind; patient is not in a position to carry out any responsible job. Weakness of the mind with weak memory. She hates people or does not like to talk with them. Patient is irritable, sad and melancholic. There is great depression of the mind, weakness of the mind. Mind is full of thoughts and ideas and there is confusion. She cannot arrive at the decision. The patient is greatly exhausted and is not in a position to think properly about any work. Physically also the patient goes weaker and weaker.

Bitter and sour taste in the oral cavity. Heartburn; acrid

eructations. Liver is tender to touch. Motions are hard and with tenesmus. Dysmenorrhoea is well marked. Nipples are hard and cracked. Itching around the pudenda; painful spasms in the stomach after eating. Dry hacking cough worse in the evening and at night. Chronic ulcers, painful axillary glands, tender to touch.

MODALITIES :

< Lying down, turning from side to side in bed, cold food, cold drinks.

> In warm room, warm food, in the dark, movement and pressure.

6.1.2 BARYTA CARBONICA

Inflammation, induration and enlargement are the fundamental pathogeneses of this drug. The mammary gland is enlarged and there is a lump, which is hard. This is very sensitive to touch. The glands which are enlarged are tender with infiltration. The women of late twenties are affected. These patients present with hard but not serrated mass with firm rubbery consistency. Their edges are sharply defined. Most commonly the tumours solitary, or occasionally are multiple. They are differentiated from cancer by smooth rather than irregular lobulations. A bloody discharge from nipple is indication of this drug. All the glands of the body are very sensitive to cold and they are worse by taking cold. The skin over the gland becomes ulcerated. It is seen that this remedy works better in Paget's disease of nipple which is supposed to be primary carcinoma of the mammary gland.

Patient is timid with weak memory. She cannot comprehend. She is afraid of strangers. Fails to remember the names of different people and location their residences. Childish behaviour of the patient. Mental development is slower than the physical. The complaints are worse when patient thinks of her disease. The patient is not in a position to remember the things as her mental growth is not up to the mark. Patient is mentally dwarfish, milestones and developments are delayed. Not in a position to concentrate her mind. Brain-fag from mental exertion.

Crackling and flapping noise in ears. Sickly, old looking face. Patient is lean and emaciated. All the glands near the cervical region are enlarged. Sore throat, inflammation of the tonsillar glands. Spasm of the oesophagus. Cannot swallow. Digestion is weak. Pain in the abdomen after eating. Distension of the abdomen. Constipation, stools are hard and knotty.

MODALITIES :

< Cold, extremes of cold, thinking of her complaints; cold drinks; cold food; change of weather.

> Open air.

6.1.3 HYDRASTIS CANADENSIS

These patients have the tendency to indurated glands. Swelling of the mammary glands. Fat necrosis and glandular cell myoblastoma are common in this remedy. Fat necrosis tumour is probably post-traumatic. Patient complains of pain and tenderness. The lesion is fixed to the breast tissue, which sometimes causes dimpling of the overlying skin. Engorged nipples, cracks and discharge of watery fluid or there is serosanguinous discharge.

The patient is weak and emaciated, fainting due to improper assimilation or defective assimilation. All - gone sensation or empty feeling in the stomach, not relieved by eating. Chronic catarrhal condition of the membrane of the stomach. Patient is thirstless. Obstinate constipation, colicky and crampy pain in the abdomen. Liver is enlarged and tender.

MODALITIES :

< Warm food, touch, pressure, heat of sun, movement.

> Rest, open air.

6.1.4 IODINE

This remedy predominantly acts on the enlargement of the mammary glands which may be either neo-plastic or malignant. The mucous membranes of the glands and the breast tissue are inflamed. The breast tissues are hypertrophied, enlarged, hard and nodular. Emaciation of the patient due to malabsorption. The tumours are well differentiated. They have a discrete capsule. Small lesions present leaf-like intracanalicular protrusions and large lesions have cystic space. Inflammation of the lesions, ulceration occasionally, excoriating and acrid discharge from the nipple or from the lesion. Oedematous swelling of the affected breast.

Patient has violent impulse to murder without any cause. She is very much anxious. Forgetfulness, weakness of the mind and weak memory. Forgets the things to carry with her. Mental diversion. Anxious and restless; wants to keep herself busy.

The patient is always hungry and wants to eat all the time which is followed by diarrhoea and vomiting. Indigestion with sour eructations. Liver and spleen are enlarged and palpable. Cough with difficulty in breathing. Heart is hypertrophied. Sense of constriction in the heart region.

MODALITIES :

< Warmth, exertion.

> After eating, cold, doing something, walking.

6.1.5 CALCAREA CARBONICA

Breasts are hot and swollen. Chronic cystic mastitis. Blunt duct adenosis; best remedy for fibroadenoma. Lump in breast is hard, nodular and tender to touch in the beginning. Then the pains are reduced and the lump turns to be hard due to calcification. Calcarea acts best when the tumours are calcified. These breasts are swollen and tender before menses. Deficient lactation. The breasts are distended in lymphatic women. Patient complains of profuse sweating around the genitalia with dirty smell Inflammatory condition of the breast.

With breast condition patient has the mental symptoms due to sufferings. Patient is anxious, tired and weak, both mentally and physically. Hysterical state of mind due to grief and exertion. The patient is sad, low-spirited and melancholic. Due to confused state of mind there is loss of sleep, insomnia. Patient is worried that somebody will observe her confused mental condition.

Headache associated with breast condition. Nausea and vomiting which makes the patient weak. Constant profuse leucorrhoea which is thick and acrid. Burning at the genital area. The glands around the cervical region are enlarged and tender.

MODALITIES :

< Cold, cold weather, cold in any form, mental or physical exertion.

> Dry climate, hot dry weather.

6.1.6 CALCAREA FLUORICA

This remedy is indicated in the fibroadenoma of the breast. Lump in the breast which is hard, movable with clear margins which are sharp in nature, or their edges are sharply defined. Most commonly they are solitary, very rarely multiple. Occurs in young patients usually unmarried. Nodules are in upper right quadrants.

The patient is sad and depressed due to financial condition. Confused due to melancholic condition of mind.

Patient is chilly, and she is very sensitive to cold air, cold wind and cold atmosphere in general. Genitals are sore. Urine is copious and offensive. Pain at the tip of the urethra while urinating and after the act. Pain in back extending to sacrum.

MODALITIES :

< Cold, cold drinks, cold air, damp weather or change of weather.

> Warmth in general, hot drinks, covering, lying on painful side.

H This remedy acts well after surgery on the breast. H

6.1.7 LAPIS ALBUS

The main action of this remedy is on the glands of mammary region. These glands have the tendency to turn malignant. Remarkable results are observed in scrofulous condition of the glands. Fibroid tumours, intense burning pains in the parts. The tumours have pliability and a kind of softness rather than hardness. The margins are not clear. The glands have elasticity, exactly the reverse of Calc. fluorica.

The skin over the lesions have got the tendency to form scrofulous abscesses, which are sore in nature. Enlargement and induration of the regional lymph nodes. Among breast conditions, cervical lymphadenitis is common.

Persistent pain in mammary region. Glandular hardening in breast region. Suppurative otitis media, changing in nature. Multiple lipomas all over the body.

Other important remedies for Tumours of Breast are

1. CALCAREA IOD.
2. CALENDULA
3. PHYTOLACCA
4. THUJA
5. PHOSPHORUS

==========

TOPIC 2

MASTITIS

6.2.1 GRAPHITES

The skin over the breast is rough and hard. Dryness of the skin near areola. The skin eruptions are itching and associated with exudate, which is watery and transparent. Frequently progresses to suppuration. In lactating cases, the patient suffers from mastitis in the very first month. The discharges from the ulcers on the breast are thin and sticky. There is swelling and induration of the axillary lymph nodes. The inflammation has tendency to form fibroma. There are fissures and cracks on the nipples and areola, which are very tender and sensitive. Hard cicatrices appear after mammary abscesses. This results in suppression of the milk flow. There is herpetic eruptions on the breast.

Along with the mastitis there are eczematous and herpetic eruptions on various parts of the body such as ears, around the anus, folds of the joints and so on. The skin eruptions or infections have no tendency to heal. Every little injury suppurates. The nails are brittle and deformed. There is excoriation between the fingers. Syphilitic ulcers are best treated by this remedy. Eruptions on the scalp with loss of hair. Patient is constipated with hard, large and knotty stool. Nausea, fulness and hardness of abdomen due to excessive flatulence. Due to distension of abdomen patient must loosen her clothings. Rumbling in abdomen with various signs of indigestion. Intense pain in stomach with temporary relief by eating, warm drinks, especially milk. Burning and stinging pains in pit of stomach.

Patient is timid, not in a position to take decision. She is fearful and apprehensive. Grief is in the background of majority of illnesses. She has changeable mood. She can remember the past events but forgets the recent ones. Music makes her weep. She has funny sensation as if a cobweb is over her face and she tries to brush it off. She is sad and despondent. Hot patient.

MODALITIES :

< Warmth in general, in the evening, at night, at the time of menstrual discharges.

> By covering, dark, cool place.

6.2.2 APIS MELLIFICA

Apis patient has a typical sore, sensitive skin of the breast. She presents classical signs of acute inflammation of breast tissue. There are stinging pains in the mammary region with sensitiveness and swelling. Burning sensation of the nipples. Hardness of the breast with erysipelatous inflammation. Oedema of breasts with suppression of menses. Sometimes there is continuous metrorrhagia which is associated with profuse bleeding and sense of heaviness in the abdomen. There is bearing down sensation when menses are about to appear. Neuralgic pains in the right ovary.

Oedematous swelling on the abdominal wall. Stinging pains in eyes, redness with hot lachrymation. Piercing pains around the orbits. Fiery red tongue. Patient is extremely thirstless and has craving for milk. She has sensation as if anus is wide open. Burning and soreness at the time of micturition. She passes little quantity of urine which is dark yellow or umber coloured. Bag-like swelling of the lower eyelid is seen. There is incontinence of urine and great burning and smarting at the end of micturition. Hot patient.

Patient has great apathy. She is awkward and loses concentration, thus drops things from hand. Confused state of mind. Cannot think properly, cannot take decisions. Jealous and frightful. Grief makes her life miserable. Unable to remember the things which she has read. Unrefreshing sleep. Dreams of flying.

MODALITIES :

< Heat in general, warm room, from getting wet in rain, touch, pressure.

> Open air, by uncovering, cold bathing.

6.2.3 PHYTOLACCA

There is mastitis with enlarged axillary lymph nodes. This mastitis is secondary to pyogenic infections. Mastitis occurs due to engorgement with milk in the early days of lactation, where one of the lactiferous ducts becomes blocked with epithelial debris. Due to this pathology, the breasts become indurated and tender. There are papular and pustular eruptions on the mammary region which have no tendency to heal. There are squamous and syphilitic eruptions on the breasts. The nipples are hard, red and tender to touch. She does not allow to touch the parts.

Soreness and intense pains in breasts. Restlessness due to inflammation is the general guiding symptom of Phytolacca even though it is mentioned that Hypericum is a glandular remedy. These engorgements of lymph nodes are secondary to local inflammation of the breast. Inflammation of the pharynx and tonsillar glands. The right hypochondriac region is inflamed and sore. Burning, griping pains in the stomach. Shooting pains in the right shoulder with signs and symptoms of frozen shoulder. Pains in legs, so severe that she has no courage to get up.

Mentally she is off and restless and has loss of self-confidence. She has great disregard for surrounding objects. She is indifferent to her own life.

MODALITIES :

< Damp wet weather, in rainy season, while moving about, at night, right side.

> Warmth in general, rest.

6.2.4 BRYONIA ALBA

This is very useful remedy for breast affections like inflammation and first stage of abscess. Breasts are very hot and stony hard. There is sensation as if the breasts are very heavy like stone. Skin of breast may be either red or pale. Stitching and tearing pains in the breasts. These pains are worse by any movement and are relieved when she is at rest. Cough also causes aggravation of both breast pain and chest pain. She has to support the breasts while coughing, moving or even while standing. Pains are worse by touch but better by hard pressure.

With mastitis, she has painful menstruation; spasmodic dysmenorrhoea. During menses ovaritis causes tenderness of ovarian region. Burning pains in the uterus. Exposure to any heat causes suppression of menses. Amenorrhoea with scanty urine. Pain in the hypogastrium and breasts. Bryonia is suitable for inflammation of breasts or sometimes heat, heaviness and hardness prior to menstruation. There is dry, hacking cough as if chest would burst from coughing. She has to sit up and then to support the chest. Haemoptysis; vicarious menstruation, nasal bleeding instead of menses. Complaints of Bryonia come slowly, steadily increase in severity and have the tendency to last longer. Hot patient.

She is very sad and depressed. Restlessness due to anxiety. She has fear of death. Demands many things but refuses when offered as she does not know her need exactly. Wants to go home even though the patient is at home. Irritability due to pains. She desires cold drinks and sweet things. She is drowsy; delirious condition. Wants to sleep all the time.

MODALITIES :

< Warmth in general, hot applications, slightest motion of the breast, touch, in the morning.

> Lying down on affected side, by supporting the breasts, cold application.

6.2.5 PULSATILLA

Mastitis of young girls due to mechanical pressure is best treated by this remedy. Local irritation which is commonly produced from too tight elastic brassiers. The affected breast presents the classical signs of acute inflammation. There is one more category where mastitis is present secondary to milk engorgement. This usually occurs at about weaning time and also in the early days of lactation. The aetiological factor majority of times is blocking of lactiferous ducts with epithelial debris. This blocking causes induration and tenderness of that particular quadrant. Discharges from breasts are thick, bland and greenish yellow. Pain associated with chilliness. Shifting pains, relieved by pressure and lying on affected side. Shooting pains. Wandering and stitching pains.

Patient has dyspepsia. Dry mouth and dry tongue without thirst. Pain in stomach after about an hour of intake of food. Thick, profuse, yellow, bland discharges characterise this remedy. Menses are suppressed from getting feet wet and nervous debility. Leucorrhoea is acrid and burning. Backache after leucorrhoea. Diarrhoea during or after menses is again a characteristic symptom. Changeability of the symptoms. All-gone sensation in the stomach in morning. Venous engorgement causes throbbing, pressive type of pains in the breast region. Tongue is cracked; lower lip cracked in the middle. Tongue feels too broad and too large.

MODALITIES :

< Warmth in general, warmth of room, after taking food, in the evening.

> Open air, moving about, cold application, cold food or drinks, consolation.

6.2.6 SULPHUR

Inflammation of Sulphur patient is very typical. Tissues get affected in the subcutaneous level. The inflammation spreads over the affected quadrant from nipples to periphery. Many a time the tissues get indurated and very rarely there is pus formation. Therefore this remedy has the symptom "threatened suppuration". Eruptions on the breast, especially the vesicular or pustular, result in mastitis. The skin over the breast is dirty looking and there is intense itching with or without eruptions. Very sensitive to touch, even the touch of cloth. This remedy has a power to establish the various types of suppurating cavities, small and large abscesses in subcutaneous level in the breast tissue. The suppurative tendency is well marked in Sulphur. The breasts get inflamed and go into suppurative condition. There is intense burning and itching of the affected breast. There is congestion and burning pain in the skin with the sensation of heat in the skin. There is irresistible desire to scratch.

She is dull and confused. She has religious mania and melancholy. Foolish ideas are prominent in her mind. She is very selfish and jealous without any gratitude. Philosophical mania, thinks of the things which have no possible answer. She is very forgetful. Thinks rags are beautiful. Aversion to business. She is very lazy. Irritable and depressed.

MODALITIES :

< While standing, warmth of bed, after washing the parts.

> In warm weather, moving about.

6.2.7 SECALE COR

Secale cor. lady has violent inflammation of the breasts. Burning pain and this burning is aggravated by heat. There are multiple eruptions around the breast. These eruptions in turn create abscesses. There is discharge of green pus from these abscesses. There is purplish appearance of affected breast with boils which contain greenish pus. The affected breast burns like fire. Horrible, offensive bloody discharges from the affected breast. In young adult patients breasts are not developed properly. Suppression of milk after confinement is seen in Secale cor. patient.

Patient is anxious. She feels and fears that death is certain and she is suffering from fatal disease and it is difficult for her to recover. Impending evil.

MODALITIES :

< Heat, warmth in general, covering.

> Cold in general, by keeping the parts uncovered.

Other useful remedies for mastitis are

1. LAC CANINUM
2. HEPAR SULPH
3. SILICEA
4. CROTON TIGLIUM
5. SABADILLA

****

CHAPTER 7

GENERAL CONDITIONS

TOPIC 1

CLIMAXIS [MENOPAUSE]

7.1.1 LACHESIS

At the climacteric Lachesis lady complains of profound prostration with palpitation. Flushes of heat. Feels the vertex, palms and the soles are hot. Recurrent attacks of headache. Emotional disturbances after slightest exertion of mind. Inflammation of glands and cellular tissues. The parts turn black and veins become varicose. The face is purple and the head is hot. Unwarranted jealousy and suspicion. Apprehension of the future. Weight and pressure on the pelvic organs. She has bursting type of headache . Sensation as if all the blood in the body is running to head. Vision becomes very intense. Oversensitiveness of auditory meatus. Warm drinks are hurtful to her stomach causing nausea. Suffocation which also increases palpitation. She has tendency to ulceration. Ulceration of those parts of skin where the circulation becomes very feeble.

The abdomen is distended with flatus. Abdomen is so sensitive that she cannot bear any clothing around the abdomen. Inflammation of the small intestine, ovaries and uterus. Pain in the left ovarian region or going from left to right. Pains in the pelvic region going upwards to the chest. Menses become very scanty and about to cease. Labour-like pains during menses. The menopausal symptoms are violent before and after flow. They are relieved during the flow. She has fainting spells with uterine haemorrhage. Suffocation in warm room. Varicosity of veins everywhere and the calf muscles are very sensitive to touch but relieved by hard pressure.

MODALITIES :

< Before and after sleep, left side, warm room, morning.

> Cold in general, flow of discharges.

7.1.2 GRAPHITES

It is the most useful remedy for the patients of climacteric age group. Where there is tendency to gain weight and deposition of fat on thighs, buttocks and around the breasts. Face is pale, waxy and sickly looking. She has aversion to coition because of the dryness of vagina. Ovaries are enlarged and hard. Great tenderness in the uterine region and both the fornices. Bearing down sensation in the uterine region. Cauliflower-like growth on cervix, uterus and vagina. Due to this overgrowth, there is burning pain in genitalia with putrid bloody discharge. Menses are late or discontinued. If appear, are irregular, scanty, pale or mixed with dark and small clots and are of short duration. Menses are about 6-8 weeks apart. Many a time leucorrhoea appears instead of menses. Oedema of the vulval region. Dryness and heat in vagina alternates with coldness of vagina. She has very much laxity during menses. Symptoms like dry cough, copious sweat, oedema on feet, hoarseness of voice, headache, nausea appear during menses. Morning nausea is well marked. Violent itching of the vulva before menses. Leucorrhoea is offensive, whitish yellow, appears instead of menses.

She is timid, confused, cannot take decisions. Lack of disposition for work. Fidgety. She has great apprehension. Despondency. Sensation of cobweb on forehead.

MODALITIES :

< Warmth, at night, during and after menstruation.

> In dark, from wrapping up.

7.1.3 NATRUM MUR

Nat. mur. lady during the period of menopause is very much emaciated and hysterical. Her skin is pale, shiny and looks as if greased. There is history of debilitating diseases like diabetes, anaemia etc. Nervous affections tremble the whole body and also there is fluttering of heart. Pulsation shakes the body. Intermittent pulse with sensation of coldness in heart. During climacteric, there is wasting of breasts. Menses become irregular. Feels hot during menses. Cannot bear hot climate, warmth of the room. The face is sickly looking and covered with vesicular eruptions. Pain in the extremities and in the muscles, are of stitching type, like an electric shock, associated with convulsive jerking of the limbs. She has a feeling as if limbs were falling asleep. Twitching of single part with shooting pains. At the time of menopause, she has oversensitiveness, becomes oversensitive to minute incidences. Intense excitability. Very emotional. The menses become too scanty. The discharges are very characteristic—thick, whitish like white of an egg. The menses are copious, scanty and watery.

Patient is thirsty and she has an unquenchable thirst for cold water; patient feels better by taking cold water. Nat. mur. lady is hot patient. She has funny feeling of lump in stomach. After taking food there is fullness and distension of abdomen. This distension and pressure on the stomach is better by vomiting. White frothy coating on the tongue. Patient is hungry. Eats well yet loses fat. She has cutting pains in the abdomen. Bleeding per rectum. Anus is contracted, mucous membrane is cracked and bleeds while defecating. Periodicity is well marked. All the complaints are worse at particular time or day. Backache, spine is very sensitive and painful. The pains are more after exerting pressure over spine. Backache is worse at the time of menses and better by pressing and by lying on something hard. Oedema of the foot.

Patient is sensitive to every change of weather. She is nervous, sad and melancholic . Hysterical condition of mind, is marked at the time of menopause. Weeping disposition. Dislikes consolation, as consolation aggravates her symptoms.

Patient is worse from sunrise to sunset, especially between 10-11 a.m. Not in a position to digest or assimilate common salt but there is intense craving for it.

MODALITIES :

< Sunrise to sunset, between 10-11 a.m., heat of sun, at the sea shore, music, noise, mental excitement, warmth in general, consolation.

> Open air, lying on hard surface, moderate exertion in cold air.

7.1.4 CALCAREA CARBONICA

All the symptoms of Calc. carb patient are due to her inability to digest or assimilate the lime which is present in her food. Thus this lack of extraction of lime from food and assimilation causes lot of physical disturbances during menopause. Mal-assimilation of calcium causes emaciation of the muscles, anaemic condition and pale sickly looking complexion of the face. There is burning and smarting in the lower extremities. Bleeding and oozing due to relaxed blood vessels. During the stage of menopause lady develops tendency of putting up weight and excessive fat. Due to this excessive fat there is increased sweating in various parts of the body even though the patient is chilly. She thinks that her heart is weak and feels weakness all over the body. Thus muscles lose the ability of to sustain prolonged efforts. She remembers the amount of work she has done before the climacteric and now feels helpless as she is unable to perform even half of that work.

She has tendency to enlargement of the glands with polypoid growths. Enlarged nasal polyp and exostosis. She is very sensitive to cold air, cold wind and every change of weather from warm to cold. There is congestion of head and also sensitiveness of both the temporals. Fat, fair, flabby and anaemic ladies with pale, waxy look, call for this remedy. Menses are scanty and they are suppressed. Constant, profuse leucorrhoea. Discharges are thick, acrid and burning. Rheumatic and gouty pains appear at the time of menopause. These pains are worse due to cold weather, cold wind and at night. Perspiration is sour smelling.

Patient is mentally exhausted due to long-lasting mental exertion. She is unable to sustain prolonged mental operations. Cannot use her brain for longer time and soon becomes tired mentally. Anxious. Fears people will look at her and would watch her mental confusion. Talks to herself. Sits in the bed or lies in the bed when alone. Forgetful and obstinate ladies. Fear of death, palpitation.

MODALITIES :

< Cold in general, wet weather, mental or physical work.

> Dry weather, lying on painful side.

7.1.5 IGNATIA

Ignatia lady is very afraid to go to bed when she passes the course of climacteric stage as there is jerking of limbs when she goes to sleep. Various dreams which makes the sleep disturbed. The menses become irregular. Bleeding is black and there are severe spasmodic pains during menses. There is prolapse of rectum as she has desire to pass stools often. Severe headache, which is of congestive type, ameliorated by warmth application. Headache increases with close attention. During menstrual period the face is distorted, convulsed, pale and sickly looking.

MODALITIES :

< In the cold, grief, anger, emotions, mental excitement, excess of stimulations.

> Warmth in general, walking in open air, after pressure.

7.1.6 SILICEA

Sick headache associated with nausea and even sometimes vomiting during climacteric period is the characteristic symptom of Silicea patient. Headache commences in the occipital region, extends forward in the afternoon and settles at the supra-orbital region in the early night hours. She has profuse head sweat which is cold, clammy, offensive, especially on forehead. Sweat on upper part of the body is the striking feature of this remedy. Silicea lady has tendency to produce inflammation and abscesses with deposition of fibrous tissue. Old ulcers heal with fibroid deposition. Many of her complaints are due to suppression of discharges, suppressed sweat. She has tendency to develop warty growths on skin with moist eruptions. The complaints of Silicea lady during menopausal period are associated with hardened glands especially about the neck, salivary glands, parotid glands. She has sickly, anaemic, waxy and tired looking face. Pustular and vesicular eruptions all over the face. The teeth break down and lose their enamel surface. She is disturbed by extremes of heat and cold; easily affected in little changes of temperature. Waterbrash with chilliness, brown tongue. Nausea and vomiting of whatever is drunk, worse in the morning. Water tastes bad is the keynote of Silicea. She has also pain in stomach and bowels. Pains are more on pressure. Abdominal pains are relieved by warm application or heat. Abdominal distension with flatulency. The lady is constipated, stools are hard and remain in rectum. Partly expelled and partly recede back. She has to strain much at stool which causes her weakness and exhaustion. Stools are sometimes removed mechanically. She has prostrated condition of sexual functions. Serous cysts in the vagina. Bloody discharges in between the periods. Many times there is absence of the menses for months together. Leucorrhoea is profuse, acrid, corroding, milky; preceded by cutting around the navel, causing biting pains.

She has yielding disposition but has fixed ideas. Pin-mania is prominent, afraid of them. She is nervous and excitable. Very sensitive to external impressions.

MODALITIES :

< In the morning, after washing the parts, while uncovering, lying down, damp, wet weather, cold atmosphere.

> Warmth in general, tight bandages around the head, in summer season, humid atmosphere.

7.1.7 SULPHUR

More suitable to a lady who leads sedentary life and suffers from the problems due to improper digestion. This indigestion at menopause changes her constitution as lean, thin and stoop-shouldered subject who walks stooping. Sulphur lady manifests the menopausal syndrome in its peculiar way. She has intense burning everywhere in body accompanied with itching. Burning is present from vertex to soles. Itching is temporarily relieved by scratching but it leads to bleeding and then there is more itching and burning. There are flushes of heat in the body. Menses are irregular, short and trouble-some. The intermenstrual period is prolonged every time and then there occurs cessation of the menses. But there is another condition also where sudden stoppage of menses occurs. In such cases violent and aggravated symptoms are observed in this patient. Leucorrhoea and menses are acrid and make the parts excoriated.

Burning and redness of vaginal orifice. Headache appears before menses. Burning and itching of nipples and breasts. Nipples are ulcerated, cracked and fissured. Pubic hair and the skin around genitalia is dry and hard. There is either anorexia or canine hunger with intense craving for sweets. She does not like milk. Weak, empty, all-gone sensation in the stomach especially at 11.a.m. Patient drinks much but eats very little due to menopausal dyspepsia. Great flatulence in abdomen and she feels that there is something live moving in abdomen or she is pregnant. Liver affections like jaundice with soreness of hypochondriac region and bilious vomiting. She has characteristic painless morning diarrhoea, alternating with constipation. Though she takes water internally she has great dislike for washing. Nocturnal, offensive sweating especially of single parts as face, nape of neck or genitalia. Standing is the worst position for her. Midnight dyspnoea with aggravation of her general condition in the morning and by warmth.

Lady at menopause behaves like a child, less power to think and is depressed. She becomes irritable and forgetful.

Patient is very selfish and having no regard for others. She is busy all the time.

MODALITIES :

< Warmth of bed, bathing, standing, in the morning [11 a.m] at rest, after eating.

> Lying on right side, dry warm weather, open air.

Other useful remedies for menopausal syndrome or climaxis are

1. PULSATILLA
2. SANGUINARIA
3. GELSEMIUM
4. APIS MELLIFICA
5. USTILAGO

* * * * * *

TOPIC 2
PELVIC ABSCESS, CELLULITIS

7.2.1 APIS MELLIFICA

The cellular tissues are inflamed and oedematous. Inflammation of the labia, vagina and the vaginal mucous membrane with stinging pain. Parts are sore and tender to touch. The pelvic peritoneum becomes inflammed and congested with lymph exudate on the surface. Due to these inflamatory signs there may be suppression of the menses. Oophoritis with severe tenderness in the pouch of Douglas. Due to severe pain in abdomen and pressure on the pelvic organs there is incontinence of urine with great irritation of parts. She complains of increased frequency of urination. Inflammation of ovary with stinging pains. Right sided ovary is usually affected. These recurrent infections of pelvic organs may lead to diseases like ovarian tumours and malignancy.

Metrorrhagia; profuse bleeding per vagina which is dark red in colour with severe pains and heaviness in the abdomen. Congestive type of dysmenorrhoea is well treated by this remedy. There is sense of tightness in the pelvic region. She has feeling as if everything is protruding out - sense of prolapse. She has pale, oedematous and waxy skin which is very sensitive to touch. Burning and stinging pains associated with soreness of the parts which suddenly migrate from one region to another indicate this remedy. Apis is thirstless remedy. She has no desire to take water except during chill stage before fever due to the pelvic abscesses. She has marked bag-like swelling under lower eyelids.

Patient is hasty, awkward and drops things while

handling. She is indifferent. She has weeping tendency. Loses courage very often. Revengeful. She has delirium especially after suppression of skin disease. Dreams of flying. There is typical sense of dryness of the skin.

MODALITIES :

< In warm room, summer season, hot application, by touch, right side, pressure, tight clothings around the waist.

> Open air, by removing the cloths and covering on body, cold application in general, by change of position.

7.2.2 MEDORRHINUM

Pelvic abscess as a result of sexually transmitted diseases or due to septic abortion. In this case, within the pouch of Douglas, the pelvic abscess is isolated from general peritoneal cavity. If not treated in time this abscess may burst into any of the surrounding hollow viscera, usually the rectum. Patient gives history of infection; injured cervix may be after obstetric operation or cervical dilatation. There may be adhesions of the surrounding organs such as ovaries, fallopian tubes, omentum etc. due to chronic inflammation. On palpation the thickened mass can be felt in right or left pelvic region. The abscess contains thick pus. Inguinal lymph nodes are enlarged.

Patient is malnourished, weak and emaciated due to long-lasting suppressed gonorrhoeal infection. She has sycosis in the background. Thus there is tendency to outgrowths, overgrowths and the malignant changes. She has metrorrhagia or sometimes she complains of menorrhagia. Bleeding is profuse which lasts for longer period and the blood is dark in colour. The blood clots very easily. Recurrent attacks of urinary tract infection. Intense burning at the tip of urethra. Burning of the soles and palms. She has ravenous hunger immediately after eating with great thirst. She complains of constipation and the stool passes in the form of small balls.

She has very irritable mind. Irritable at every trifle. She wants to do everything in a hurry and hastily. Thus she gets exhausted very early. She is very forgetful as there is great weakness of memory. She has very peculiar weeping tendency and it is very difficult for her to narrate the symptoms without weeping. Anxious about her day to day activites. Anticipation is found in Medorrhinum patient. She even anticipates her death.

MODALITIES :

< In daytime, i.e. from sunrise to sunset, thinking of her complaints, by warm application, heat of sun, by covering the parts, by motion.

> In damp wet weather, lying on stomach, at the seashore.

7.2.3 RHUS TOXICODENDRON

Rhus tox. lady complains of violent inflammation of the bowels. This intestinal inflammation may be secondary to typhoid fever or associated with typhoid condition. Very likely there may be perforation of the intestine at Peyer's patches. This results in general peritonitis. Sometimes there may be acute inflammation of appendix and if not treated properly it may burst to create a condition of general peritonitis. There is intense pain in abdomen especially in right iliac fossa and in pelvic cavity. Inflammation of the uterus, the tubes and the ovaries. There is violent tenesmus in the pelvic region due to pelvic abscess.

The skin in flushed. She has violent thirst and wants to drink often. She also complains of pain in the stomach with nausea. Distended abdomen due to pelvic inflammatory condition. She has great urge to urinate with tenesmus in the region of bladder neck. There is sense of incomplete evacuation due to recurrent pelvic infection and pelvic abscesses. The supports of the uterus have lost their normal strength. Therefore there is great weakness of all the pelvic muscles. Menses are irregular and copious. Blood is clotted, therefore labour-like pain during the periods. She also complains of inflammation of the lungs. There is severe stupifying headache. Great restlessness; erysipelas of the face with burning. Tongue has red triangular tip with imprints of teeth. There may be fever associated with pelvic pathology which is intermittent or continous in nature.

Patient is extremely restless and wants to change position very often to find comfort. She is sad. She has fear that somebody will poison her. She has delirious condition. She has typical dreams of her day-to-day activities.

MODALITIES :

< Right side of the body, cold wet or damp wet weather, first motion.

> Slow continuous motion, dry weather, by hot application.

7.2.4 BRYONIA ALBA

Rheumatism and typhoid fever create gastro-hepatic complications and the patient may land into peritonitis. She has tension in liver region with stitching pains. Abdominal walls are very tender. Oophoritis with stitching pains in the region of right ovary. Pains are more when there is increased intra-abdominal pressure. Pains extend to thigh and she feels as if the ovarian region is torn. Skin above the swelling is dry, red and hot or pale. Heaviness and stony hardness of the abscess is marked. There are stitching and violent throbbing pains in the abscess. Pelvic abscesses are associated with mammary abscess. Pelvic abscess leads to menstrual disturbances like menorrhagia, dysmenorrhoea or amenorrhoea. Pelvic region feels too sore and the pains are relieved by hard pressure and cold air. Motion also aggravates her condition.

Constant motion of left arm and leg. In general the patient is very hot and has dryness, heat and tenderness everywhere. Mouth is also very dry and she drinks large quantities of water at longer intervals. The mucous membrane of bowels is also dry so she has obstinate constipation. The stool is dry and hard, looks as if burnt. Acrid and offensive diarrhoea. Tendency to dropsical effusions in the serous cavities.

Bryonia lady is forgetful, depressed and anxious. She gets easily excited and is ill-humoured. During fever she has delirious condition of mind. She wants to go home though she is at home. Constantly talks about the daily routine or business.

MODALITIES :

< Exertion, heat of sun, warmth, touch, motion.

> Rest, hard pressure, lying on affected side.

7.2.5 SILICEA

Silicea has got both internal and external abscesses. The lady has labial and internal pelvic abscesses too. Inflammation of the pelvic viscera leads to suppuration, there forms an abscess. History of gonococcal infection. The related discharges are cadaveric smelling or offensive. Pelvic abscesses may lead to intermenstrual bleeding. Polymenorrhoea. There are attacks of icy coldness of whole body. Offensive milky and acrid leucorrhoea. Discharge of pus is grey, gelatinous and foetid smelling. Pulsations in the abscess with burning and pricking pains.

Silicea lady is very chilly and easily disturbed by cold weather. Rachitic lady with scrofula. Chronic constipation with receding of the dry and hard stools after partially expelled. Stools are foetid. Constipation before, during and after menses. Skin is pale and thin with waxy appearance. Abscesses after vaccination. History of malnutrition or chronic infections of pelvic organs. Sweat on foot, palms, axillae, behind neck and in the occipital region is very offensive. She may also present with lump in breast. Haematuria with involuntary micturition. There are abscesses and boils everywhere. Headache when the stomach is empty. Intense photophobia. Somnambulism.

Mentally Silicea lady is anxious, nervous and obstinate. Brainfag in obstinate ladies. Pin mania. She has fixed ideas in her mind. Hypersensitive. Reacts quickly to any impressions.

MODALITIES :

< Washing, cold in general, during menses, uncovering.

> Covering, warmth in general.

7.2.6 CALCAREA CARBONICA

This remedy is useful in both pelvic cellulitis and pelvic abscess. The lady has tendency to form abscesses in the deeper parts especially in the muscle tissues. Uterine outgrowth and easy displacement of uterus. Before the menses she has chilliness with uterine colic and leucorrhoea. Leucorrhoea is milky, acrid and causes pruritus. Due to abscess the menses are altered as too early, too profuse and these last too long. She has cold sweating on feet. Hot and swollen breasts during menses due to endocrinal effect. There are cutting and colicky pains in abdomen. Great flatulence. Abdomen is very tender. Mesenteric and inguinal lymphadenopathy. Abdomen is very distended and feels too hard. She cannot bear any touch of the abdominal skin. Constipation. At first the stool is dry, hard and large, then it becomes semisolid and then liquid.

Rheumatic affections of various joints, major as well as minor. There is sense of weakness and she is easily fatigued. The perspiration is smelling very sour. Along with abscesses she has tendency to form polypi and exostosis also. She is very chilly and catches cold easily. Sour taste in mouth with foetid smell. Palpitation with sensation of coldness. Cramps in the pelvic area, stomach and muscles of extremities due to the underlying abscesses.

Calcarea carb lady has aversion to mental or physical exertion. She is very confused, anxious, headstrong and forgetful. She fears of losing reason and also about misfortune. Marked apprehension is also observed. Restlessness, great irritability and sadness.

< Washing with cold water, touch, cold air, wet atmosphere.

> Pressure, dry weather.

7.2.7 HEPAR SULPHURIS CALCAREUM

Whenever there is an abscess formation, it is limited by an external tumour. In Hepar patient the tumour has pricking and burning pains. These abscesses bleed very easily. Pelvic abscess with affection of uterus mainly. Chronic abdominal or pelvic ailments cause tension in that region. Metrorrhagia. Leucorrhoea is putrid and smell like old cheese. The menses are too late to appear and the discharge is very less. Abscesses are formed also in the regional pelvic lymph glands. Always worse in cold air and relieved by warmth as the patient is chilly, wants covering. Perspiration does not ameliorate her troubles.

Hepar lady has also tendency to form glandular swellings. In other regions, it produces chronic catarrhal inflammation causing copious exudate. Gets chilled easily and aphonia or hoarseness of voice. Also useful in hepatic abscesses. Dribbling of urine due to atonic bladder. Stool is soft but rectum has no power to expel it and so she feels constipated. The superficial absceses spread by forming multiple small papules around them. She feels as if wind is blowing over some parts. Splinter-like pains in the affected parts.

Hepar lady is hypersensitive and becomes irritable at every trifle. She has great hastiness in her every act. Destructive tendency with violent impulses. Anxiety and sadness. Anxious in the evening and towards night.

MODALITIES :

< Cold air, cold in general, uncovering, touch, pressure, dry weather.

> Warmth in general, covering, damp wet weather.

Other useful remedies which for pelvic abscess are

1. MERC. SOL.
2. LACHESIS
3. CORTALUS HORRIDUS
4. BELLADONNA
5. SULPHUR

=========

TOPIC 3
BACKACHE

7.3.1 KALI BICHROMICUM

Stabbing pain in back which is of rheumatic type. They are sharp, shooting in nature. Pains shift up and down. In left side from scapular region to hip. Pains in coccyx. Cutting pains in loins, shifting, the patient has difficulty to walk. Pains fly rapidly from one place to another. The pains of Kali bich. are wandering along the bones. Worse in cold atmosphere. There is affection of lumbar vertebrae, usually L4, L5, which causes pressure symptoms and results into left sided sciatica. Bones feel sore and bruised. Tearing pains in muscles of the back. Backache associated with joint pains where there is swelling and stiffness. There is crackling sound in joints during movement. Pain in tendo-achillis region, which is swollen and painful. Pain in small spots that can be covered with the tip of finger is a characteristic symptom of Kali bich.

Constant twitching of a group of muscles. Patient is thirsty and she has constant hiccough. Jerking and twitching of the muscles of abdomen. She has neuralgic pain in the ovaries with great restlessness. Ovarian tumour along with backache is well treated. Gastric symptoms are worse in summer. Digestion is weak. Leucorrhoea is yellow and stringy. Menses are early and excoriating, causes burning of the parts. Sticky, stringy discharges which adhere to the underparts and can be drawn in long strings. Backache is worse from motion and comes periodically, for instance at the same time everyday. Patient is greatly prostrated, tired of life, with cold sweat especially after the pains or when the complaints are passed off.

MODALITIES :

< In the morning, cold weather, cold atmosphere.

> Lying down, pressure.

7.3.2 CIMICIFUGA

Upper and lower cervical vertebrae are usually affected. They are very tender to touch. Pain in the cervical region extends downwards to back. Soreness with bruised feeling all over the body. The muscles of the back are stiff. Spine is very sensitive. Stiffness and contraction in the nape of neck and back is very common of this remedy. The intercostal muscles go into spasm causing dyspnoea. Rheumatic pains in the muscles of back, in lumbosacral region and these pains, travel down the hips and thighs. This causes restless feeling in hips. Heaviness of lower extremities with tensive pains.

Cimicifuga lady has profuse menses which are dark, coagulated, offensive and always associated with backache. Pain in back immediately before menses. Pains across the pelvis from hip to hip. Shooting and throbbing pains in the head. Nausea and vomiting caused by pressure on the stomach and pressure on the spine and cervical region. Sinking in epigastric region. Patient is sleepless, irritation of brain; wild feeling in the brain.

Sensation of a cloud enveloping her. Mental symptoms alternate with rheumatism; worse after menses. Those women who call for Cimicifuga are hysterical or in puerperal mania. She thinks that she will go mad and tries to injure herself. She is very much depressed, sad and fearful.

MODALITIES :

$<$ Before menses, cold air, cold application.

$>$ Warmth in general.

7.3.3 AMMONIUM MUR.

This lady complains of bruised and sprained sensation in between the scapulae with feeling as if the skin were stretched tight. Icy coldness between the shoulders not relieved by warm covering. These pains in the back are followed by itching. Bruised pains in coccyx when sitting. Shooting and tearing from back to lower extremities. Backache often wakes her from sleep. Joints are oedematous and cracking noise in all the joints. Neuralgic pains in the extremities make the patient unable to walk. Thus cannot she walk erect.

Hoarseness and burning in larynx. Dry, hacking cough which is worse lying on back . Abdominal symptoms appear during pregnancy. Chronic congestion of liver. Menses are too early, profuse and the blood is dark, clotted. Flow more at night times. Haemorrhoids after suppressed leucorrhoea.

Patient is melancholic. She has great apprehension, probably from internal grief. Desires to cry but cannot do so. Bad consequences of suppression of grief.

MODALITIES :

< In morning, after walking.

> Open air.

7.3.4 CARBOLIC ACID

Patient has great sense of weight in the cervical region with tenderness on touch to that particular region. Pains are terrible, come and go suddenly. Physical exertion makes the pains more. Soreness in the muscles of back which extends to lower extremities. The soreness is so severe that she can hardly make her legs straight. Cramps in the legs and in the tibial region especially during walking. She is prostrated and tired out from least exertion.

Patient does not like mental work. Tight feeling as if compression around the head. Nervous.

MODALITIES :

< By riding and movement.

> Rest.

7.3.5 ARNICA MONTANA

Lumbago from overexertion and straining. Backache results from blow, fall, blunt trauma and mechanical injuries. Pains are sore, lame and bruised with great sensitiveness to pressure. If the backache results from contusion or trauma then the affected part becomes blue and black due to extravasation of blood. Pressive pains between the scapulae with crawling in vertebral column. Cutting thrust extending to chest while walking. Paretic and paralytic condition of the parts. She has ascending type of rheumatism from sacrum to cervical region. She cannot bear the pains. Cannot walk erect on account of bruised pains in cervical region.

Sore, lame, bruised feeling all over the body as if beaten is the characteristic of Arnica. It is suited to cases where injury is on the background of present complaints. Everything on which the patient lies, seems too hard. Sprains and dislocations are set right by this remedy. She has foetid breath. Mouth is dry and thirsty. Canine hunger. Pain in the stomach during eating. Sleepless and restless when she is overtired.

MODALITIES :

< Least touch, motion, rest, damp cold weather.

> By lying down in head low position.

7.3.6 AESCULUS HIPPOCASTANUM

Backache of Aesculus lady is always associated with the haemorrhoids. There is fulness of various parts along with the muscular, rheumatic pains. Marked paralytic feeling in the back or spine. Back gives out and makes the patient unfit for any work. Weakness, weariness and lameness is more in the lumbar region. Constant dull backache across hips and sacrum. In morning the patient is unable to sit in the bed. Intense aching between the scapulae with lameness in the nape of neck. Backache is more when she stoops or walks or even turns in the bed.

Other important complaints which are associated with backache of the Aesculus ladies are the haemorrhoids and bleeding per rectum. There is sense of fulness in the rectum as from several small sticks. Prolapse of rectum at climaxis. Left sided renal and ureteric colic with frequency of micturition. Pulsations all over the body with sense of constriction around chest. Hepatic congestion may cause reflex cough.

Lameness and tired feeling in limbs with darting and shooting pains. The lady also complains of constant throbbing behind symphysis pubis. Leucorrhoea with lameness of back, lameness across the sacro-iliac articulation. Leucorrhoea is worse after menses. Dryness of nose and throat; the veins in throat are varicosed. Throat is very sensitive and feels scalded. Burning and fulness in stomach so she has intense desire to vomit after eating. Violent occipital headache, dull in nature, more in frontal region and starting on right side traverses to left side. Patient is sad and depressed due to various physical ailments. There is great confusion of mind and loss of memory. Increased sexual desire. She is very irritable and loses self-control even for small causes.

MODALITIES :

< Morning, eating, sleep, motion.

> Cold, open air.

7.3.7 RHUS TOXICODENDRON

Mainly useful in the rheumatic pains of back, may be due to straining, sexual excess or exposure to cold, damp weather. Constrictive pains in the back while sitting. Soreness and lameness all over with bruised feeling. Pain between scapulae while swallowing, with tension. Rheumatic stiffness is affecting the nape of neck after strain, overlifting. Uterine troubles lead to spinal irritation. Sensation of burning in loins with contusive pains in lumbar region. Pain in cervical muscles. Patient is aggravated at rest and by change of position. Continuous motion ameliorates the pains but later on the patient feels exhausted and tired.

This drug may be indicated in typhoid state. During febrile condition she is very restless. Dry cough with urticaria and other eruptions. Stiffness of pelvic joints with pruritus vulvae and oedema of genitalia. Trembling and palpitation at rest. Protracted lochia. Catarrhal condition of eyes, nose and ears from getting wet in rain or from suppressed sweat. Redness of tip of tongue; rest part is coated. Fever blisters around the mouth with intense dryness in mouth. Patient has unquenchable thirst with bloody saliva. Putrid and metallic taste. Vomiting of bilious substance. Numbness and feeling of paralysis of the limbs with urticarial rash during fever.

MODALITIES :

< At rest, change of position, after mental work, cold, damp, wet weather, getting wet, before a thunderstorm, night, open air.

> Change of position, dry weather, rubbing, warm application, motion, stretching out the limbs.

Other important remedies for backache are

1) PHOSPHORUS
2) NUX VOMICA
3) PULSATILLA
4) BRYONIA
5) NATRUM MURIATICUM

===============

CHAPTER 8

OBSTETRIC THERAPEUTICS

TOPIC 1

ABORTION

8.1.1 CAULOPHYLLUM

Caulophyllum is known to cause relaxation of the muscles of uterus, cervical os and atonicity of the uterus. Therefore the patient gives history of habitual abortion or miscarriage. She also has amenorrhoea for about three months with vaginal bleeding. Blood oozes out for want of tonicity. Passive haemorrhage. Severe pains in back and loins with spotting indicate threatened abortion. Uterine contractions are abnormal therefore products of conception cannot be retained up to normal growth or full term. Uterine debility with incompetent os. Passive lochia oozes out for days together. Relaxation of muscles and ligaments. Excoriating leucorrohea. The products of conception are thrown out with only slight loss of blood.

Lady presents the history of early or delayed menses. Rheumatic pains are mainly of tearing and drawing type. Rheumatism of small joints of limbs. Neck region and fingers are stiff with migrating or shifting pains. Chorea of young girl with delayed menarche. She is very sensitive to cold and suffers from rheumatism. She always likes to remain warm.

Patient is very much hysterial, fearful and apprehensive. The pains make her sleepless, restless and very irritable.

MODALITIES :

< Cold, open air.

> Warmth in general..

8.1.2 CHAMOMILLA

Chamomilla is indicated in threatened abortion resulting from anger or mental distress. She has irregular contractions of the uterus with cutting and tearing pains which bring out the products of conception. If she has psoric condition, the products of conception remain until first trimester but the same may act as exciting cause for habitual abortion. Severe backache; labour-like pains, begin at back and then travel to the medial aspect of thighs. Great nervous excitement. Discharges of Chamomilla lady are very typical. They are profuse and clotted. Blood is dark red in colour. Spasmodic pains cause downward pressure on the uterus. Inflammatory condition of the endometrium due to infection. Yellow acrid leucorrhoea with tearing pains at the time of abortion. She has great nervous excitement with discharge of dark offensive blood. Increased frequency of micturition.

Patient is very sensitive to pains and she cannot bear these intolerable pains. Pains are more during heat and make her very exhausted. The parts are made numb. She is very sleepy but she cannot sleep due to pains. Patient is over-sensitive to open air but longs for it. One cheek is red and hot while other is pale and cold. Convulsions; rheumatic pains.

Mentally the patient is very restless and cannot bear anybody and herself too. Fretful and impatient, mannerless, spiteful; wants things but refuses when offered. Doesnot like to talk or to listen. Answering in cross and in childish manner. Has no regard for emotions of others. Very irritable and loses temper easily.

MODALITIES :

< Evening, early night, open air, heat.

> Warm wet weather, passive motion.

8.1.3 PULSATILLA

Threatened abortion is well treated by this remedy. Blood flow is thick and in the form of clots but there is changeability of this flow. The character of the blood changes. The blood flows, stops and again starts flowing. Intermittent flow, serum and blood clots are separated. There is milky white leucorrhoea which is acrid and burning but painless. As changeability is marked, once again these characters of leucorrhoea may change. Vesicular moles are expelled by this remedy. Sexual desire unusually strong during this period. History of suppression of gonorrhoea or STD. She gives history of suppression of menses from getting feet wet. Pains in the pelvic region come suddenly or go gradually or come insidiously and go suddenly. Soreness in the uterine region.

Patient has very much striking and peculiar totality of symptoms. All discharges of Pulsatilla lady except leucorrhoea are bland and yellowish green. Only the leucorrhoea is acrid and milky or cream-like. The pains are associated with chill. More the pains, the chills are also more. Pains are aching and flying from one site to another. Thirstlessness with dry tongue. She has all-gone feeling in stomach or sometimes stony heaviness. Night diarrhoea.

Mentally she is very emotional and has weeping tendency but may change to happy and joyful mood suddenly. Yielding disposition, gentle females. Fear of darkness, opposite sex and ghosts. Consolation ameliorates her troubles, at the same time she has sympathy for suffering of others.

MODALITIES :

< Warmth in general, evening, night, feet hanging down.

> Cold in general, pressure, open air, motion, consolation.

8.1.4 SABINA

Sabina is indicated for the abortion during third month. It is useful in the patients having early menarche with tendency to miscarriage. Severe shooting pains from back to pubic symphysis with sense of bearing down. Typical labour-like pains at the time of abortion. The discharges of blood during abortion are watery and sometimes copious, bright red and clotted. Products of conception are mixed with partly clotted blood. Inflammation of the uterus, ovaries and fallopian tubes after abortion. There are violent pains from ovary to uterus. Ovarian neuralgia during abortion is well treated by this remedy. Severe, violent, throbbing, tearing pains with profuse bleeding indicate this remedy. More bleeding after motion, better at rest.

Peculiar manifestation of sycosis by skin outgrowths, rheumatism, gout and nervousness of mind. The figwarts or condylomata are intensely itching and burning. Nodosities and swelling of the joints with shooting pains and joints are red. In Sabina lady gouty complaints are alternating with the bleeding. Feels tired and is anaemic due to haemorrhages. Shaking of whole body with each pulsation. Drawing pains.

Music is unbearable and she becomes sad due to it.

MODALITIES :

< Warmth in general, motion.

> Fresh and cool open air.

8.1.5 BELLADONNA

Violent, shooting pains in the uterus with sudden gush of blood from the uterine cavity calls for Belladonna. There is inflammation of endometrium and other accessory genital organs due to secondary infection. This leads to expulsion of the products of conception. Sudden and violent bleeding without any warning sign is well marked. Pressing type of pains from uterus to vulva as if the uterus will be pressed out from vagina. Severe backache as if the bones are broken down. Discharge of bright red blood with high degree of fever. Throbbing in the womb. Septic abortions. Discharges of blood are hot and the parts are sore and inflamed.

Belladonna has got heavy congestion of the upper parts of the body and those are hot with shiny red colour. Burning and dryness of mouth, yet she has no thirst during fever. No sweat. Throbbing pains in the affected parts.

Patient has violence and delirium due to cerebral

hyperaemia. Very impulsive and excited easily. Offending everybody. Fear of imaginary things. She uses vulgar words in speech and tears the clothings. Unconsciousness.

MODALITIES :

< After 3 p.m., midnight, heat, touch, motion, external stimulus.

> In warm room, standing erect, lying down.

8.1.6 SECALE COR.

Threatened abortion is well treated by this remedy. Amenorrhoea of about 3 months. Discharges of black and non-coagulable blood. Severe pain in abdomen prior to blood flow. In other words the abdominal pain after 3 months of amenorrhoea associated with blood flow indicates Secale cor. She gives history of irregular menses. Copious watery blood flow, prolonged until next period. The parts are relaxed therefore the products are thrown out. After abortion there is high degree of fever. Dark, offensive lochia. Due to prolonged discharges the parts are cold and pulse is feeble. Tingling and numbness in extremities with violent cramps in calf muscles. Intense burning pain in the uterus. Brownish offensive leucorrhoea.

Externally there is chilliness with internal burning. Passive haemorrhages exhaust her and make her very anaemic and marasmic. Atonicity and weakness of muscles with cramps. Craves acid or sour thing. Dislikes fat and meat which are heavy to digest for her.

Anguish, fear of water with suicided impulses. Tendency to bite in maniac ladies. Unconsciousness.

MODALITIES :

< Heat, touch, warmth in general.

> Cold in general, open air, massage, cold applications.

8.1.7 SEPIA

Habitual abortions especially from 5th to 7th month of gestation. Sense of heaviness in the abdomen with relaxation of pelvic organs. Bearing down sensation in the pelvic organs.

Cervical os is dilated therefore products of conception are out. Stitching pains from vagina to uterus. All the signs of pregnancy in first trimester but as the gestation advances, products are expelled out. There are flushes of heat with sense of faintness. Profuse, dark coloured bleeding. Painful sensation of emptiness in the uterine region with indurated os. Leucorrhoea is yellowish, greenish and acrid in nature, it causes soreness of genitalia.

Weakness with relaxation of the parts. Pains settle in the back. Patient has low vitality so tendancy to catch cold. Faints at sudden change of weather. Great aversion to smell or sight of food, it nauseates her. Desire for spicy food, but dislike of tobacco and meat. Milk in pregnant lady causes diarrhoea. Foul smelling breath. Obstinate constipation due to paretic bowels. Skin is showing various eruptions.

Anaemic condition with dyspnoea. It is ameliorated by moving slowly or dancing but is aggravated by taking complete rest. All-gone sensation everywhere with bearing down pains.

Mentally anxious and depressed. Sad and weeping or tearful mood, she cannot narrate without weeping. Feels that she is helpless so becomes irritable. Consolation aggravates the mental disturbances and makes excited. Fearful, fear of opposite sex and being alone. She has marked indifference to herself and others. She is also indifferent to her occupation and domestic problems. No desire to do anything or to think too.

MODALITIES :

< Dampness, cold air, morning and evening, night.

> Warmth, cold bathing, pressure, rest, exercise.

Other useful remedies for abortion are

1) PYROGEN
2) CALCAREA CARBONICA
3) MERC COR.
4) HELONIAS
5) VIBURNUM OPULUS

TOPIC 2

ANTENATAL CARE

8.2.1 ARSENICUM ALBUM

Arsenicum album has great role in the antenatal care of women who complain of painful distension of abdomen. Violent, burning pains. Appetite is lost. Complaint of hiccough after eating and the food is vomited out. Vomiting usually at night times with green or black water. She has thirst for cold water. Disturbances of stomach from taking ice-cold things, over-ripe fruits, etc. She has desire to pass stools after eating. All the troubles are marked in the first trimester. Burning pain in the epigastric region along with sensation of heaviness. Loathing of food. Vomits as soon as food reaches the stomach. Profound weakness and debility. Leucorrhoea in the first trimester is very marked in Arsenic. It is profuse, yellow, thick and corroding which is offensive in nature. Constant sense of exhaustion. Pressive, stitching pains in the right ovarian region which extends to right thigh. Burning pains in the breast and breasts are tender to touch.

Pain about the umbilical region, makes her to bend forward. She has painful, spasmodic protrusion of rectum. Intense burning in the anus after defecation. There is trembling of extremities with ineffectual urge to pass stool. Sometimes involuntary stools which are black in colour. Burning in the mouth with excessive thirst. Wants to drink cold water but is afraid to take it, as it is vomited out soon. Bitter taste in mouth. Dyspepsia; ulceration of the oral cavity due to improper assimilation. Involuntary urination. Scanty urine. Palpitation with dyspnoea. Swelling of feet. Sleep is disturbed, therefore drowsy all the while.

MODALITIES :

< Wet weather, mid-day, mid-night, over-ripe fruits, cold in general, smell or sight of food.

> From heat in general, warm drinks.

2.2 COCCULUS INDICUS

She complains of continuous vomiting and thus unable to retain anything. During the early weeks of pregnancy the protein hormones such as HCG (Human Chorionic Gonadotrophin), HPL (Human Placental Lactogen), HCT (Human Chorionic Thyrotrophin) etc. are secreted by placenta. The lady is hypersensitive to these proteins therefore a kind of reaction takes place. She vomits in large quantity which includes undigested food particles. There are violent cramps in the stomach with griping pain. Nausea with faintness. There is great distension of abdomen but has a sense of emptiness and hollowness. There is pinching and constrictive pain in epigastric region which increased on deep inspiration. There is dryness in oesophageal region with hiccough. She desires cold drinks, as cold drinks give relief to her. Excessive nausea as soon as she gets up in the morning. Therefore she has scareto rise. Colicky pain in the abdomen usually at mid-night with passing of flatus which give very little relief.

She has extreme aversion for food especially sour things. She feels better by taking cold drinks. She has unusual nausea and vomiting in the early weeks of pregnancy termed as hyperemesis gravidarum. In other words Cocculus indicus is the remedy of choice in hyperemesis gravidarum. She has leucorrhoea which is like serum. She complains of pressure on the uterus causing much pain. She has a peculiar constrictive tension on the right side of the chest on inspiration, with nervous palpitation of the heart. She complains of stiffness of all the joints which are painful. Trembling of extremities. Due to constant vomiting, she has great weakness. It is difficult for her to stand firmly due to this weakness. Muscular power is reduced. She has unrefreshing sleep due to night watching, due to anxiety and restlessness.

She is sad and thinks of bad part of the matter. She pays very little attention to her day-to-day activities. Constantly thinks about her sickness. Due to these complaints she is very irritable. She thinks that she has committed great mistake. She cannot tolerate any contradiction. Thinks that time is passing too quickly.

MODALITIES :

< From eating, after drinking, while going to bed, while riding in a carriage.

> Bending forward.

8.2.3 NATRUM SULPHURICUM

During early weeks of pregnancy all the systems of body undergo physiological changes. On fertilisation of the ovum, the effect of increased progesterone is seen on the body. This increased progesterone level disturbs the cardiac function and also the respiratory system. It acts upon the respiratory centres to cause overbreathing and consequently pulmonary ventilation rises. The gums may become vascular. There is increased frequency of urination. She complains of duodenal catarrh with sharp stitching pain in the region of duodenum with increased flatulency. Constant bruised pain in the rectal region. Vulval region is hypersensitive and there is secondary herpetic eruption of the vulva. She has yellowish green leucorrhoea with hoarseness of voice. Due to this progesterone disbalance, she has dyspnoea. She has to support the chest while coughing. She has intense burning in the abdomen. This burning is increased even after taking small amount of water. She has violent occipital pain and vertigo in the first trimester.

Asthma during pregnancy is well treated by this remedy. She has rattling in the chest usually early in the morning. Cough associated with greenish, thick expectoration which is ropy or sticky. She has to sit up in the bed as cough increases. She has inflammatory condition with oedema of joints. Burning pains in soles with oedema on feet. She has a strange feeling of heat on the vertex. She has dreams of running water. Itching of the parts with watery blisters.

She is melancholic with history of repeated attacks of mania. Suicidal tendency is well marked in Nat sulph lady. Due to various physiological changes going on in the body, she is unable to think and thus dislikes to be spoken to.

MODALITIES :

< Lying in the bed, music which makes her uneasy, damp wet weather.

> Dry weather, change in position.

8.2.4 PULSATILLA NIGRICANS

Pulsatilla is useful in all the complaints from which the females usually suffer during pregnancy. The pains of Pulsatilla are of shooting type and they are always changing their places. If these pains are more, then she feels more chilly. These pains are marked in the nape of neck, between scapulae and in the lower back. Bitter taste in mouth with waterbrash and there is offensive smell in mouth. Mouth is dry, then also she has no thirst and the saliva tastes sweet. Retrosternal burning pain with indigestion. There is sense of weight in abdomen with severe pain after taking food. Complaints of hiccough after smoking. Alteration of the taste. Obstinate constipation. Leucorrhoea may be thick or thin and it is milky or creamy. It is the only excoriating acrid discharge in the patient. Drawing, tearing pains in the limbs with deathly coldness. From head to toes there are jerking and drawing pains. Weakness of feet.

The Pulsatilla lady has got peculiar and characteristic general complaints. There is marked changeability in every ailment. No two complaints are similar. When they re-appear, they always change their character, location or other features. Nearly all complaints are accompanied with chill. More the chill means symptoms are aggravated. All the discharges of the Pulsatilla lady are bland except the leucorrhoea. She has diarrhoea only in nights. Intense desire for fatty food and tonics. She has aversion to bread, milk, curds and butter. Irresistible desire to sleep in afternoon. During night she is sleepless. Tired feeling in the evening.

Mentally the Pulsatilla lady is timid, gentle and amiable. Though she has yielding disposition, she is very emotional. She is easily discouraged with slight ailments. Fear of opposite sex. Hypochondriac. Mental picture of Pulsatilla is always changing from one extreme to the other.

MODALITIES :

< Heat in general, evening, pregnancy, fatty rich food, warm room.

> Cold in general, open air, movement and pressure.

8.2.5 NUX VOMICA

Nux Vomica is known for its extreme irritability and excitability everywhere in the body and in the mind too. In the morning there is vertigo and loss of conciousness during vertigo. Tickling in the throat. Mouth is dry and she has not much thirst but due to profuse and bloody saliva there is bad taste in mouth. In the morning and after taking food she complains of nausea and bitter taste in mouth. She feels that she will be better only after vomiting and so she tries to vomit but fails to do so. She desires stimulants and fatty food. Marked dyspepsia. Fluttering in the epigastrium. Flatulency. Colic is spasmodic and creates upward pressure and thus shortness of breath. The abdominal skin is bruised and feels sore. Alternate constipation and diarrhoea. Constriction of the rectum so there is frequent desire for stool. But it comes to be ineffectual and there is a feeling that some part has remained. The lady also suffers from convulsions due to her hypersensitivity. There is tetanic rigidity of all the muscles. Violent, contractive pains with great weariness. She wants to sit or lie down. Sleepy in the evening. Loud respiration in sleep.

In general the lady is emaciated, lean, thin and oversensitive. She has got sedentary habits and has congestion or stasis of portal system. Photophobia and otalgia from loud sounds. Nose runs only during day but stuffs up at night. There is sense of loss of power in limbs with cracking in joints when walking. The gastric trouble causes headache and skin eruptions. Face is burning hot. Backache or lumbago more when sitting. Drowsy after meals. Chilliness when uncovered but she does not like to be covered.

Nux vomica patient is hypersentive and over-impressionable. Cannot bear any stimulus. Very irritable and spiteful. Fault finding nature. Sensation as if time passes too slowly.

MODALITIES :

< Any external stimulus, overeating, morning, cold air.

> In damp, wet weather, rest or lying down, evening, pressure.

8.2.6 NATRUM MURIATICUM

There is extreme debility and feeling of prostration while she is in the bed in morning. She is exhausted both mentally and physically. Pulsations even at rest and it shakes the whole body. Loss of taste, frothy coating on tongue. Unquenchable thirst and desire for salt. Though she eats well she loses flesh. Awareness of heartbeat. Sweating when she takes food. Retrosternal burning pains after taking food. Irresistible desire to sleep in the forenoon. She has dreams of robbers and she wakes up and searches every corner of the house and then sleeps again. Weakness, trembling of the extremities. Palms are hot and have much sweat. Nervous jerking of limbs during sleep. Backache with desire to rest the back on some firm thing. Cramps in left foot. Headache is only during daytime. Increased intra-abdominal pressure causes frequency of urination due to pressure on bladder. Relaxation of bladder muscles causes stress incontinence. Stasis of the urine may cause infection. Discharge of mucus from urethra. There are cutting and burning pains in urethra after micturition. Pressure on lumbar and sacral plexuses causes cramps in the leg muscles. Dry, hard stools difficult to expel and cause burning and stitching pain in anus. Thus constipation may cause fissures in anus.

During pregnancy instead of weight gain there may be cachexia and prostration. She has intense craving for salt, milk and fish. Aversion to coffee and tobacco. Alopecia; hangnails; various skin eruptions. All the complaints are worse during daytime, i.e. from sunrise to sunset. Extreme aggravation of headache at 10 a.m. It is also useful when there is pregnancy in an anaemic woman. Sense of sticking in the throat excites cough. Tinnitus.

Mentally she is very awkward and hasty. Lachrymation when she laughs. Depressed but extremely irritable. Desire to cry. Consolation aggravates her mental and general symptoms.

MODALITIES :

< When lying down, at seashore, heat in general, daytime (10 a.m.), mental work.

> Lying on right side, pushing back against firm support, cold bath, open air, meals at daytime.

8.2.7 SILICEA

Silicea lady suffers from imperfect assimilation of food material, therefore suffers from defective nutrition. Constipation is frequent ailment of pregnancy. Delayed emptying of bowel is due to diminished tone of the muscles of the intestines. This is thought to be due to effect of progesterone. Silicea lady complains of paralysis of the rectal muscles. There is painful spasm of the sphincter. Stools come down with difficulty and recede back when partly expelled. In first trimester, there are cramps of back muscles. Her spine is weak. Pain through coccyx and hips, legs and feet. Piles get aggravated in pregnancy due to constipation. Cramps in legs, more during night. Cervical secretion is increased. Nipples are sore. Incontinence of urine. Sometimes increased frequency at night times. She has to rush for urination when there is desire or otherwise urine dribbles in clothings. Nauseating sensation with painful cold feeling in the pit of stomach. Various metabolic deficiencies are noted in Silicea patient. She has poor weight gain during pregnancy. It is well marked in first trimester.

Recurrent attacks of cold and she has tendency to catch cold very easily. Cough with sore throat; expectoration in the form of small granules or sago-like particles. When crushed, smell very offensively. Cough is more on lying, skin is dry. Complains of eczemaious erruptions on the skin. Abscesses in joints. Patient has obstinate constipation and she has to strain for defecation. Leucorrhoea is milky white and it is usually at the time of urination. There is intense itching of genitalia with burning and soreness.

Patient is obstinate. She is very sensitive to external impressions and cannot tolerate the words against her performance. She has tendency to think over the expressions or the opinions of others; results in brainfag. She has fixed ideas and she is firm about her ideas. She has funny thinking about pins and is afraid of the pins.

MODALITIES :

< Cold in general, after uncovering, when lying down.

> Warmth in general, summer season, damp wet weather.

Other useful remedies for antenatal care are

1) FERRUM METALLICUM
2) CICUTA VIROSA
3) RHUS TOXICODENDRON
4) PULSATILA
5) CALCAREA CARBONICA

==========

TOPIC 3

ANTEPARTUM HAEMORRHAGE

8.3.1 ARNICA MONTANA

Profuse haemorrhage of bright red colour mixed with clots, due to premature detachment of placenta from uterus. Arnica is sometimes indicated in traumatic APH. Mechanical trauma due to forceful external cephalic version, fall, traction of the umbilical cord during labour as it is short. The uterus is soft and it is prolapsed. Profuse haemorrhage with pain in small of back extending up to groin and down the medial side of thighs. Pulse is feeble, great dryness of mouth, vertigo, when she bleeds.

Arnica patient is very sensitive to pains. She feels hot in upper parts of body while lower parts are cold. She has sore, lame, bruised feeling everywhere and she feels that her body is beaten by something. Every surface on which she lies feels very hard and it causes pains. Bleeding is mainly internal and there may be extravasation of blood under skin. Rheumatic pains are ascending. She cannot walk in erect position.

Patient is absent-minded and wants to be alone. Fear of being struck by everybody who approches her. She is having delirious condition; loss of consciousness.

MODALITIES :

< Rest, touch, motion, damp, wet climate.

> Lying down.

8.3.2 CAULOPHYLLUM

Passive haemorrhage before the labour starts. Bleeding from lax uterine cavity. Weakness felt all over the body associated with the blood flow. Sense of exertion and drowsiness. Retroplacental bleeding followed by the compression of inferior vena cava by gravid uterus. It causes sudden onset of haemorrhage. Followed by profuse bleeding, she delivers hastily. As the uterus remains lax the blood vessels remain dilated and APH goes on. The labour is delayed due to want of contraction or due to rigid os. Thus the quantity of blood loss again increases. Very important factor in Caulophyllum is the inertia of the uterus with relaxation of uterine muscles and ligaments.

Useful remedy in the complaints of female during parturition and lactation etc. Gouty diathesis of lady with muscular rheumatism. Passive haemorrhage. She is always exhausted and there is lack of power in every system. Inflammation of small joints. Drawing and tearing pains with stiffness of muscles. Joints are swollen. Ptosis of upper eyelid.

MODALITIES :

< Coffee, in open air.

> By passing flatus.

8.3.3 CROCUS SATIVA

Patient is not in labour but there are mild pains in the abdomen. Dark clotted blood flows in long strings. APH from overloading of the uterine vessels and thus there is passive congestion. Profuse bleeding which is dark, seedy and viscid in nature. Bleeding starts after overlifting or from straining. Uterine haemorrhage after full term with jerking indicates Crocus sativa. There are cutting pains deep in lower abdomen extending to back. During haemorrhage the feet are icy cold. Patient has sense of fainting with palpitation. Full bounding pulse; jerking pains in the interior of left breast. Sensation of something alive in the breast. Colicky pain in abdomen during haemorrhage. There is spasmodic contraction of a group of muscles and there occurs twitching of single muscle. Sensation of something alive moving in hollow visceral parts. Chorea.

Patient has got changing mental conditions and moods.

She becomes angry and spiteful then becomes happy and affectionate. Sometimes she may weep. Usually very joyful and happy lady. Hysteria and hallucinations.

MODALITIES :

< Warm room, hot summer, rest.

> Moving in open air.

8.3.4 FERRUM PHOS

It is one of the great anti-haemorrhagic remedy. APH with copious discharge of partly fluid, partly black and coagulated blood. There is bearing down sensation and pain in the uterine region. These patients have tendency for prolapse of uterus. The supports of uterus are relaxed. Vaginal bleeding is severe and continuous. Patient becomes pale and anaemic with coldness of extremities. Many times the haemorrhagic blood collects between the placenta and the uterine wall and quantity of the blood cannot be determined. But as the blood pressure lowers down and pulse becomes fast from this, concealed haemorrhage may be diagnosed. Thus it is to be kept in mind that in pale, anaemic subjects with violent local congestions and profuse vaginal bleeding which is bright red in colour before delivery, Ferrum phos is the remedy.

Lady is having false plethora and she flushes easily on every excitement. But she is originally too anaemic. Bright red blood from every orifice. She is very prostrated. Due to anaemia more prone to get chest infections and has dyspnoea on least exertion. Frequency of urination. Urine comes out when there is increased intra-abdominal pressure. Involuntary urination during sleep at night. Tachycardia, awareness of her own heart beats; congestion of head. Craves stimulants and has dislike for meat and milk. Watery stools. Patient is anxious and restless. She has dreams of anxiety and is sleepless due to the same.

MODALITIES :

< Right side, touch, jar, motion, night (4 - 6 a.m.)

> Cold application.

8.3.5. SABINA

These patients have an uncomfortable feeling prior to parturition with increase of pulse rate, and drowsiness. Profuse blood flow intermingles with clots. There is pains extending between sacrum and pubis. Profuse flow lasts for longer time with increase of the foetal heart sound. Bleeding is sometimes dark. These patients are usually multiparous. They are known cases of anaemia and suffering from hypotension syndrome. The APH is excited with the slightest motion. Excessive blood flow causes severe debility and weakness. Abdominal colic. She also gives history of recurrent attacks of menorrhagia.

Skin shows figwarts and other outgrowths with intense burning and itching. May be a sufferer of gonorrhoea with sycotic tendencies. She is very hot and wants to remain in open air so keeps doors and windows always open. Easily aggravated by heat. Tearing pains in the bones and periosteum. Pains are from sacrum to pubis and are deeply aching. Music is unbearable for her, it makes her very disturbed and nervous. She feels that music passes through her bones.

MODALITIES :

< Warmth, least motion, jar, heat.

> In open air and cold air, fresh air makes her comfortable.

8.3.6 SECALE CORNUTUM

Painless profuse bleeding may be due to placenta praevia or due to defective coagulation. Due to this APH causes cortical necrosis and infarction of the decidua. The bleeding usually is slight, continuous and dark. No severe pains but feels uncomfortable. Papilloedema. Headache with vomiting is sometimes present. Pain in abdomen with coldness and intolerance of heat. Passive haemorrhage in feeble and cachectic women. Tearing pain in the uterus with copious dark bleeding. Continuous oozing of watery blood prior to parturition. During labour no expulsive action even though the cervical os is relaxed and the uterus is well contracted.

Dark offensive lochia. Patient is not in a position to pass urine during labour. On slightest motion there is severe bleeding. No expulsion of foetus but profuse haemorrhage with strong and spasmodic contraction of uterus. Every flow is preceded by strong bearing down pains.

Every affection makes her more debilitated and prostrated. Atonicity of every smooth muscle fibres leading to relaxation and weakness. Small wounds bleed profusely and the skin becomes icy cold. She has aversion to covering and likes open air. Various types of skin eruptions on the skin. Burning of all the body as from sparks of fire and is better by cold application. Tingling of the limbs with weakness. Though she looks scrawny she eats well and she drinks more.

Violence of mind, wants to bite. Fear of death and of running water. She has impulses to jump in it. She is mad with lowered sensorium; unconciousness.

MODALITIES :

< Heat in general, covering, touch.

> Cold application, open air, uncovering.

8.3.7 HAMAMELIS VIRGINICA

Congestion of the uterus and the genital tract. Also there is varicosity of the uterine vessels. This remedy is well indicated in passive venous haemorrhages. Blood is dark red in colour, passive in nature, non-coagulable and always before the expulsion of foetus. There is fullness and soreness in abdomen. Evidence of toxaemia may be present. Anaemia is observed in these ladies as they have haemorrhagic tendencies. Haemorrhage from any orifices. Placenta may not be felt at lower uterine segment but friable and soft blood clots can be felt. APH of this type is very risky for the patient, as she may suffer shock due to haemorrhage.

Throbbing pain in the stomach associated with tenderness of vagina. There are great bearing down pains in the back. Useful in all diseases of the blood vessels where there is passive haemorrhage and the bleeding parts are made sore and bruised.

All the complaints after haemorrhage are also well treated by this remedy. Pain at the tip of left shoulder and under right scapula indicate this remedy. Bleeding from nose, mouth, rectum etc. Retinal and intestinal haemorrhages. Varicose veins; haematuria.

MODALITIES :

< Warmth in general, moist air, touch, motion, afternoon, physical work.

> Open air and staying at open places.

Other useful remedies for antepartum haemorrhage are

1) ACONITUM
2) PHOSPHORUS
3) BOVISTA
4) CARBO VEG.
5) ACETIC ACID

=================

TOPIC 4

HYPEREMESIS GRAVIDARUM

8.4.1 CARBOLIC ACID

Excessive vomiting in early months of pregnancy with marked prostration. Appetite is lost. Constant belching. Due to loss of appetite patient constantly loses weight. Cramps in legs; dry tongue, brown in colour with crack. Tachycardia, pulse is soft. Vomit contains undigested food material and foul smelling liquid. Vomiting is dark, olive green. Temperature may rise in stomach. Bad taste in mouth. Constipation due to loss of body fluids. All discharges are offensive.

Patients are thin weak and prostrated. Tendency to form ulcers and carcinomas. Paralysis of the respiratory centre induces general prostration and headache etc. Vomiting is always accompanied with complaint of dysentery and stool contains large mass of mucus, it resembles the scrappings of intestines. Headache with right sided orbital neuralgia. Sensation as if the head is pressed with a very tight band around it. All discharges are very offensive. Vesicular eruptions with itching and burning. Urine is dark or black in colour. Pruritus vulva. She has aversion to strong smell. Does not like any mental work.

8.4.2 ARSENICUM ALBUM

Hyperemesis in Arsenicum album may be due to two reasons. First is the anxiousness of the patient and another is the hormonal imbalance due to pregnancy. Severe burning in the whole digestive tract. Stomach is oversensitive. Vomiting of all the food what she has taken. It has got horrible odour. Smells like cadaver. Distressing vomiting. Nausea even at smell or sight of the food. Any food or drink induces vomiting. Burning pain in the epigastric region. Frequent eructations. Gastralgia from very little quantity of food or few sips of drinks. Icy coldness of the extremities with great exhaustion. Dryness of mouth and unquenchable thirst, drinks sip by sip to moisten her mouth. Abdomen is distended and tympanic. Pain in abdomen on coughing.

Patient seems to be too much debilitated or suffering from chronic ailments. She has got peculiar cadaveric smell of her body and of all discharges. Any discharge causes more prostration. Tearing pains in bones and muscles. Skin is very senstitive to cold and cold applications. Intense burning pains are relieved by warmth. Only the head troubles are better by cold air. Generally she is worse at 1-2 a.m. or 1-2 p.m. Mostly the troubles are more after taking cold food or cold drinks. She is so exhausted that she is unable to do even little movement of her body.

Mentally she is very anxious and fearful. She fears that she has got some incurable disease and medicines are helpless to save her. Mentally restless due to anxiety. Fastidious and weak memory, forgetful.

MODALITIES :

< Cold food, cold drinks, mid-day, Mid-night.

> Warm drinks, warmth in general, raising the head.

8.4.3 PHOSPHORUS

Severe vomiting and belching. Even water is thrown off as soon as it gets warm. Nervous spasm of the cardiac opening of the stomach. Therefore anything which reaches the stomach regurgitated as the pylorus goes into spasm. Tongue is smooth, white and dry but not thickly coated. Pain and tenderness in the left hypochondriac region. Burning pains in the stomach are relieved by cold drink but it is vomited as it gets warm there. Gastritis with burning extending to throat and bowel. Desires excess of salt. Abdomen feels very cold with sharp cutting pains. Weak, empty, all-gone sensation in pit of stomach is well marked. Stools and vomitus are fetid. Cannot stand due to debility and fatigue.

Mentally the patient is very intelligent and also oversensitive. She has desire to be magnetised but she is very apathetic and indifferent to anybody. Fearful during evening and in darkness. Very sluggish in movements and thoughts. Fear of death when alone.

MODALITIES :

< During thunderstorm, evening, pressure, before mid-night.

> From being rubbed, cold drinks and cold food, in darkness, lying on right side.

8.4.4 FERRUM MET

Vomiting immediately after eating. She takes food and rushes to bathroom and takes out whatever was taken. Nausea and vomiting after eating. Eructations of food taken hours before. Sense of heat and burning in the stomach. Soreness in the abdominal wall with flatulent dyspesia. Typical tendency to spit out the food from mouth while eating. Absolute loss of appetite due to fear of vomiting. Desires sour things but when she takes these, either vomits or gets diarrhoea. Vomiting after mid-night. Does not tolerate eggs at all. She has got extreme sense of fullness in the stomach region with pressure especially after eating. Painless diarrhoea and lienteria.

Every bleeding is bright red in colour. Haemorrhages with dysmenorrhoea. Menses with tinnitus. Tongue is fiery red while the red parts become white. Complaints are worse during rest or exertion and better when she moves gently. Anaemia with canine hunger and trembling. Dropsical condition.

She is very weary and depressed. Confused mind with tearful mood. Irritable lady, despondent and anxious. Easily excited and restless from any noise. Dizziness on sudden motion. Flushed face with mental excitement.

MODALITIES :

< Rest, at night.

> Hot weather, walking slowly.

8.4.5 COCCULUS INDICUS

Nausea with faintness and large quantities of vomitus. She has aversion to food or drink. Typical metallic taste. Cramps in the stomach before and after taking meal, relieved after vomiting. Hiccough followed by regurgitation. Smell or thought of food makes the patient to gag. Bitter or sour taste in mouth. Paralysis of the oesophagus causing dysphagia. Sensation as if there is a worm in the stomach. Spasms of stomach with griping and constrictive pains. Muscular weakness and sleeplessness. Motion induces vomiting and makes her unconscious.

Great prostration of the body with sense of weakness in the parts like head, abdomen, throax. Excitement causes trembling. Leucorrhoea instead of menses.

Lassitude of mind with sluggish comprehension. Time passes too quickly. She cannot bear any contradiction. Forgetful, mental weakness.

MODALITIES :

< Sleep, smoking, motion, eating or drinking.

8.4.6 IPECACUANHA

Ipecacuanha is very useful remedy in the acute complaints and it has particular action on the stomach. First there is pain in between the shoulder blades, then it descends down the whole back. Pyrexia with shivering and she feels that her back will break. Spasmodic irritation of stomach causing colic with persistent nausea and vomiting. Clean tongue, moist mouth with no thirst. Bilious vomiting. Sensation as if the stomach is heavily loaded. Cutting colicky pains traverse from left to right. Pains cause catching of breath.

Dyspnoea, coryza and violent cough. Haemoptysis, hoarseness of voice or aphonia. Photophobia.

She is very irritable and takes everything is bad part. She desires various things but not knows what to do with them.

MODALITIES :

< Every winter, humid weather, rest.

> Motion.

8.4.7 SEPIA

All-gone sensation in the pit of stomach. She has typical hungry and empty feeling in the stomach not relieved by eating. Nausea with bulky, curd-like vomiting in the morning. Sour and bitter eructations of food. Vomiting of bile. Sour eructations. These eructations bring up acid from the stomach to oesophagus causing heartburn. Burning and stitching pains in the stomach usually after taking food. These pains are not relieved by vomiting, on the contrary they are intensified. Rumbling and gurgling in abdomen with profuse vomiting in the first trimester makes the lady too weak. Patient goes weak and emaciated with repeated vomitting as she retains very little in stomach. Severe retching and nausea is continuously present. She has constant urging for urine. The salts and electrolytes are lost by vomiting. Urine is concentrated, with burning.

Sepia lady is very chilly and she takes cold very easily. She is worse during the extremes of both heat and cold and faints due to it. Dyspnoea is worse at rest but better by dancing. Sense of heat with sweating. Feels fulness of the genital organs with bearing down. Stomach feels very empty and weak. Craves acids, sweets and dislikes tobacco, meat and even the smell of any food. It nauseates her. Yellowish discolouration of skin.

Mentally Sepia lady is known for irritability and indifference. Indifferent to occupation and domestic problems. She has very sad mood and anxiety prevails over her. Weeping tendency. Depressed and does not like to work or even to think.

MODALITIES :

< Getting wet, dampness, evening, cold air, morning.

> Warmth of bed, cold bath, hot application, pressure, exercise.

Other useful remedies for hyperemesis gravidarum are

1) ACONITUM
2) SILICEA
3) NUX VOMICA
4) LACHESIS
5) NATRUM MURIATICUM

=============

TOPIC 5
LACTATION

8.5.1 HELONIAS

Breasts of Helonias lady are very hot, swollen and painful. Nipples are cracked and fissured so she cannot feed her baby. There is intense itching and burning pain in the nipple and areola. The nipples are sensitive and she cannot bear the touch or even clothing. Prostration and low backache. Any movement aggravates the pains and she becomes irritable. Copious urine, clear in colour. She is sleepless due to the pains.

Weakness of the pelvic region. She feels prostrated at every derangement in life. Other general debilitating conditions may cause leucorrhoea. History of prolapse due to weakness of supports. Intense itching in the genital region. Muscular fatigue with burning and aching, feels as if cool wind flowing up the legs.

She is worse when alone or thinking of her complaints. So it is necessary for her to divert her attention to any other subject. She gets relief when she is busy. She cannot tolerate any opposition, irritates her. Melancholic females.

MODALITIES :

< Touch, motion.

> Mental diversion.

8.5.2 NUX VOMICA

Deficiency of milk in a nursing woman can best be treated by this remedy. Breasts are deminished in size. Nipples are dry and sore. Ducts of acini are blocked. Engorged breast on third or fourth day. Acute mastitis with rise of temperature on fourth day. Unpleasant feeling of emptiness in the breast. Pain in breast when the baby sucks.

Congestive headache and vertigo. Oversensitiveness to any impressions and gets trouble due to it. Irritable mind and body. Sensitive spine and burning along the spine. Cramps in the skeletal and smooth muscles. Weakness of extremities with sudden paralytic feeling. Nausea and vomiting in morning or some time after eating. Feels that she will be better only after vomiting but she cannot vomit. Gastric derangements due to abuse of coffee. Alternate diarrhoea and constipation. Retention of urine or involuntary urination. Urine passes drop by drop and causes pruritus.

Mentally she is very irritable and spiteful. Oversensitive and feels that time passes too slowly. Oversensitiveness of mind is marked.

MODALITIES :

< Mental exertion, dry cold weather, morning.

> Pressure, damp wet weather, at rest.

8.5.3 AETHUSA CYANAPIUM

Retracted nipples. They are very raw and sore. Baby sucks the milk but then vomits. Copious vomiting and then baby becomes exhausted. Cries sharply for feed, but cannot tolerate mother's milk. This leads to engorgement of breast and she has to drain the breast mechanically. Mother is uneasy and has discomfort. Due to this there is suppressed lactation. Lancinating pains in the breast. Mother is unable to digest food. She has nausea even when she sees food. Swelling of the breast accompanied with black spores. Nocturnal pains severe at areola.

All troubles are seen when there is extreme heat or in hot summer season. The child cannot bear milk in any form. Even mother's milk makes it to vomit.

Sensation of fullness in ears and eyes. Though there is profuse vomiting and dryness of mouth, complete absence of thirst is striking symptom. Pruritus and lancinating pains in the vulval region and breasts. Cold sweat with palpitation.

Restlessness is well-marked in Aethusa lady, idiocy and anxiety. Irritable.

MODALITIES :

< Warmth, in the evening.

> Open air.

8.5.4 GRAPHITES

Blackish, dirty coloured blisters on the nipples. The nipples are sore with corrosive ulcers on it. Discharges of colourless, sticky liquid, sometimes serum or gelatinous fluid. This fluid forms a crust on the areola, on nipples, which is difficult to remove. While removing the crust there are abrasions on the nipple. This causes lot of irritation and burning. Violent pains with suppression of the milk. Skin over the breast is rough, hard and there is persistent dryness over it. Cracks in the nipples which bleed easily with burning and stinging pains.

Graphites lady has tendency to malignancy of genital organs and mammary glands. Anaemic lady. Congestion of head. Generalised dryness of every part. Every food nauseates and she vomits it. White and acrid leucorrhoea. Offensive breath. Induration of the soft parts. Constricted feeling around chest causes asthma.

Not inclined to work but hurries to start anything. Indecisive. Despondent and apprehensive.

MODALITIES :

< Heat in general, night.

> From covering.

8.5.5 CASTOR EQUI

The nipples are cracked and sore in nursing women. Stitching pains, breasts are excessively sensitive and tender. Touch of any kind is intolerable to her. Even she cannot bear the touch of clothing. There are multiple ulcers on the breast, on the areola, with fetid discharge. The ulcers are inflamed, indurated which then turn into abscesses. From these ulcers there is stringy discharge which is bland in nature. Areola and nipples turn red like erysipelas. Usually left breast is affected with suppression of milk. Milk fever is well treated by this remedy.

Thickening of the soft tissues, later on they become ulcerated and cracks are also formed. She has also got tendency to form outgrowths like warts especially on forehead and breasts. Aching bone pains, tibia and coccyx are commonly affected.

8.5.6 OLEANDER

Breasts are engorged, hot and tender; difficult to nurse. After feeding there is sense of emptiness in the pit of stomach. This cannot be removed even after eating. This lady complains of nausea and vomiting constantly. So cannot take enough quantity of food, this results in suppression of milk. Tardy and scanty appearance of milk especially in nursing women with abdominal symptom call for this remedy. Vertigo, numbness and double vision. Itching and sensitiveness of skin. Difficult breathing. Oozing and bleeding eruptions, varicosity. Muscular affections like cramps and paralysis. Soreness of parts.

Melancholic lady. Forgetful and delayed perception due to weak memory.

MODALITIES :

< Rest, touch, uncovering.

8.5.7 PULSATILLA

Milk is thin and watery, which contains hardly any milk globule. There is sudden suppression of milk in nursing women. Lochia is milky white in nature. Breasts are swollen and engorged. It becomes very difficult for baby to suck the breast due to its sensitivity. So to prevent breast abscess, the breasts must be emptied mechanically. Pains spread all over the chest from nipple. These pains wander from place to place while nursing. There are cramps in abdomen and back while nursing.

Pulsatilla is thirstless remedy and she has got chronic dyspepsia. All-gone sensation is stomach in morning. Changeability is seen in every ailment and there is marked sensitiveness in every organ. Increased frequency of urination, colicky pain in bladder. Bland piles with blood in dysentery. Chilliness is associated with all the troubles. It increases or decreases with those ailments. All the discharges in Pulsatilla lady are bland, only acrid discharge is the leucorrhoea. It is milky or cream-like and very much offensive. Drawing and tensive pains in limbs. Pains are shifting rapidly and associated with chilliness.

She is very timid, gentle and sensitive. Weeping tendency. Has fear of the opposite sex. Fear to be alone or of darkness.

MODALITIES :

< Heat in general, left side.

> Pressure, cold.

Other important remedies for lactation are

1) BORAX
2) SILICEA
3) SULPHUR
4) PHYTOLACCA
5) PALLADIUM
6) DULCAMARA
7) PHELLANDRIUM

TOPIC 6
MORNING SICKNESS

8.6.1 PHOSPHORUS

Patient is very sleepy. She has very sensitive abdomen, painful to touch. Violent pain in the ovaries extending down the inner side of the thighs in the first trimester. Vomiting usually in the morning. She has violent palpitation, more after movements. She has neuralgic pains in the limbs. Restless due to insufficient sleep, thus patient feels drowsy in the morning. Wants to sleep in evening. She likes to eat, as many of her gastric troubles are ameliorated by eating. Cannot go to sleep until she eats something. Pain in pit of stomach with nausea and vomiting. There is burning in stomach which is ameliorated by cold things. Dislikes warm food. Nausea in the pregnancy is well treated by this remedy. She has eructations. Desire for cold water and ice, cold drinks, but vomits as soon as it gets heated in stomach. Wants something cold which refreshes momentarily. This thirst for cold drinks reappear when cold drinks get warm in the stomach. Unquenchable thirst. Dryness of mouth and throat; stomatitis or oral cavity is covered with thrush. Vertigo usually in the morning. Staggering while walking as if intoxicated. Vertigo after taking food in evening. Heaviness and confusion in head. Burning in the rectum during stool. Copious diarrhoea; constipation. Stool is hard, long and slender, like dog stools. She has no urge to pass urine though the bladder is full.

Phosphorus lady is very chilly and her complaints appear from getting wet in rain, more during the thunderstorm and evening. She is oversensitive to external stimuli. Anxious lady. Restlessness with intense burning everywhere and everytime in the body due to pathology in blood. Burning in between the shoulder blades. Nymphomania. Desire to be rubbed vigorously. Though the patient is chilly, the stomach, face and head symptoms are relieved by cold. During pregnancy, though she craves cold drinks, sight of water causes nausea and vomiting. She closes her eyes while taking bath. Perspiration smells like sulphur.

Mentally she is very keen but physically too weak. Indifferent to every person in contact. She wants to be magnetised as she has exaggerated ideas about her own importance. Sad, sluggish, tearful.

MODALITIES :

< Pressure, evening, thunderstorm.

> Rubbing, cold food, darkness.

8.6.2 ACETIC ACID

There is sour belching and vomiting during pregnancy with profuse water-brash. Excessive salivation; fermentation in stomach. She has violent burning pain in stomach and chest, followed by coldness of skin and cold sweat on forehead. Sour and bitter taste in mouth with excessive salivatiion day and night. She has constant feeling as if some ulcer is present in the stomach causing all the trouble. She vomits after every kind of food. Epigastric tenderness. Distension of abdomen after food. Nausea in the first trimester with painful enlargement of breast. Milk engorgement. Milk is bluish and transparent. Nipples are sore. Distress in stomach gives great uneasiness. She has intense thirst and passes large amount of urine, with great prostration.

She has dropsical condition of the body. Haemorrhages may cause fainting attacks and hot feeling with pulsations. Oedema of legs with ulcers on the mucous surfaces. Patient is pale, thin and having anaemic look. Uncontrollable thirst; burning and gnawing pain in the stomach with distension. Abdominal discomfort is relieved by lying on the stomach or by pressure. Rheumatism of upper and lower limbs with lameness and weak feeling.

Mentally she is very confused and peevish. Forgetful. Cannot remember the recent events and forgets her own relatives. Complains about everything. Irritability.

MODALITIES :

< Exertion.

> Rest, lying on abdomen.

8.6.3 PLATINA

Useful when selected on the basis of mental symptoms. She has got very much sexual excitement during pregnancy. Tickling and itching of the parts. Oversensitiveness of genital organs may prevent coition, vaginismus. She has obstinate constipation. Stool is very hard and dark. She has urge but she cannot pass the stools. Flatulent distension of abdomen. Sense of pressure and bearing down in abdomen. Numbness; colicky pains. Slow onset and slowly ceasing pains. Tension of scalp with pressing pains in the head and there is sense of numbness. Dragging pain in pelvis. Neuralgia of face. Haemorrhages from different parts of body and mucous outlets. Cramping pains in the limbs with numbness and trembling. Pressive pains in thighs and legs. Ravenous appetite or anorexia. Coldness of various organs. She has history of early menses which are too profuse and lasting very short. Shifting neuralgic pains with spasms, coldness and cramps.

Mentally the lady is victim of "superiority complex" and she has got "nymphomania". She thinks that she is of higher race and others are inferior to her. She has sense of growing in all directions. Alternate tearful and cheerful mood of a hysterical lady. Becomes serious over small things. Anxious and fearful. Proud of herself. Taciturn. All the mental disturbances are due to sexual excess and fright.

MODALITIES :

< In evening, night, on excitement, sitting or standing still.

> Motion, open air, cold.

8.6.4 KREOSOTUM

Kreosotum lady has got very peculiar head, stomach and extremities symptoms. Headache with dull, occipital pain and there is sensation as if a board is pressed against forehead. Deafness and tinnitus. Bitter taste in mouth with foul smell. When the lady takes food there is sense of burning in the stomach and then she nauseates and vomits within two hours. Undigested food particles are seen in vomitus. Very offensive smell. Sourness in abdomen with haematemesis. Frequent and sudden urge to urinate. Dragging backache. Arthralgia of hip joint and knee joints. Sleep is disturbed.

All the discharges of Kreosotum lady are putrid and acrid. They burn the parts upon which they pass. There are violent pulsations all over the body. There is profuse haemorrhage from small wounds. Eczema, pustules and ecchymosis. Dreams of fire and anxious events. Haemorrhoids.

Patient desires so many things but does not like them when offered and refuses those things. She is very irritable and is worse from music. It makes her weep and brings palpitation. She is very childish, stupid and has loss of memory.

MODALITIES :

< By cold in general, rest, open air.

> Motion, warm food and warmth in general.

8.6.5 PSORINUM

Useful remedy for the females especially with psoric miasm in the background. The lady has very much decreased vitality and is easily disturbed due to any changes. She has history of chronic vomiting. Ulcers. Haematemesis is also seen. Chronic diarrhoea with bloodstained stools. Offensive smell of hard, constipated stools. She is very sleepless from the itching eruptions. Sluggishness or slowness is well marked especially of bladder and bowels. Though the stool is normal she has to strain much to expel them. Though the bladder is full, she passes urine very slowly and there is feeling that some urine is retained. Least work causes palpitation, pulse is weak and rapid; arrhythmia. Eats well but does not grow. Headache with congestion of head. Head sweats profusely. Hunger at mid-night. Eructations are tasting like rotten eggs and cause nausea. She is worse when exposed to cold, open air. Throat has accumulation of profuse and fetid saliva and mucus. Leucorrhoea with lumps of mucus and having carrion-like odour.

The Psorinum lady has humid skin eruptions. Secretions are acrid and offensive. Hair dry and matted. Profuse perspiration makes her feel better and she has aversion to cold, open air. Lady gives history of suppression of skin diseases or exposure to cold air. Upper eyelids are swollen. Snuffles or dry nose. More sweating at night. Weariness of the joints. Dyspnoea on exertion, better by rest and worse in cold air and when she sits up.

Mentally, Psorinum lady is melancholic. Sadness, anxiety, fear that she will not recover from her ailment. Irritability. Hopelessness.

MODALITIES :

< Cold open air, change of weather, heat of sun.

> Warmth in general, perspiration, taking food.

8.6.6 SILICEA

Silicea lady has got scrofulous diathesis. Though the patient is chilly she wants cold food and drinks and she has aversion to hot food and drink. Canine hunger with increased thirst but the drinks cause vomiting. Frequent sour eructations after eating. Feeling of pressure at the pit of stomach. Nervous exhaustion, feels tired at night. Great aversion to milk and it induces vomiting. Waterbrash, nausea and vomiting in the morning. Brown tongue with taste of blood in mouth. Colicky pain and flatulence. Irritated sphincter ani goes into spasm. Obstinate constipation and she expells some part of stool, some part recedes back and she has to strain much to defecate. Haematuria. Pain in coccygeal region and the spine is very weak. Neuralgic pains in thighs, legs and upper extremities. Feels as if the limbs are paralysed. Cramps in legs with contraction and tension of calf muscles. Soreness of soles. Severe aching and bursting type of headache. Bruised pain above the eyes. Pain from occiput extend to vertex and then settle over right eye. Headache induces nausea and chilliness.

Very offensive perspiration of hands, feet, axillae. Head perspires profusely. Feet have carrion-like odour without any sweating. Haemorrhoids and fissures in anus. Acrid leucorrhoea; pruritus vulva. Lady has tendency to enlargement and suppuration of the glands. Assimilation of food is hampered and she has undernourished constitution though she eats well. Somnambulism. Cough when she lies down. Hoarseness with cracked voice. Cough is dry and teasing. Sputa is very fetid; stitching pains in the chest.

Irritable and nervous lady. Oversensitive to all impressions. Yielding disposition. Anxiety and fearful mind. Brainfag from overwork and dread of undertaking anything. Cross and despondent.

MODALITIES :

- < In morning , uncovering, washing, cold air, lying down, inhaling cold air.
- > In summer, warm application, wrapping the head.

8.6.7 ZINCUM METALLICUM

Slow digestion and she feels as if the stomach collapsed. She has giddiness while eating, sweet food causes heartburn. Canine hunger especially about 11 a.m. Distension and griping pain in abdomen after eating. She complains of hiccough and nausea. Vomiting mainly mucus which tastes bitter. Before nausea she has sensation as if the eyes are drown together. Dull headache with heaviness and trembling. Lumbago. Burning of spine with weariness in neck. Weakness of muscles with trembling and twitching. Constant motion of feet. Walks during sleep and there is involuntary jerking of muscles preventing sleep. Stools are small and hard. Constipation due to weakness of rectum. Coldness is everywhere and is marked.

All complaints are relieved by discharges. Hoarseness of voice with spasmodic cough. Dyspnoea with feeling of constriction of the chest and she has cutting pain in chest. Itching eruptions with varicose veins and varicose ulcers. Dysphagia due to painful pharyngeal muscles. Anaemic look of face. Expectoration relieves dyspnoea. Eats and drinks very greedily. Bleeding gums. Photophobia with redness of eyes and profuse lachrymation. Thickened eyelids. Tearing pain in facial muscles.

She is oversensitive to least noise. Stupid lady. She has very weak memory due to lethargy. Before answering she repeats the whole of what was asked. Melancholia. Feeble-minded. She has aversion to work and to talk on her favourite subject or person too. Brainfag from over-exertion.

< After dinner, touch, alcohol.

> Discharges, eruptions and while taking food.

Other useful remedies for morning sickness are

1) LACHESIS
2) ARSENICUM ALBUM
3) LOBELIA INFLATA
4) GOSSYPIUM
5) PETROLEUM

=============

TOPIC 7
LABOUR

8.7.1 GELSEMIUM

Gelsemium is indicated where there are false labour pains. There is no dilatation of the os and cervix. These pains are non-progressive. Pains running directly upwards or backwards. Lady is hypersensitive to pains. Due to these pains the patient is much exhausted. The cervical os is hard and it is not at all dilating. With every pain the foetus seems to be ascending upwards instead of downwards. There are spasmodic, intermittent, ineffectual and irregular pains in abdomen and patient thinks that those are labour pains. These severe and sharp false labour pains shoot up the back and down the hips and legs. There is another condition where the os is fully dilated but due to atony of uterus the pains are inefficient or sometimes absent. Labour is always associated with nervous chills. Soreness and bruised feeling of the abdominal walls. Dullness, dizziness and drowsiness along with nervous trembling. Loss of muscular power to contract effectively and expel the foetus. So it is more useful in delayed labour either due to rigid cervical os or poor uterine contractions.

Congestion of the trunk and head only. They become hot while the extremities are very cold. Chills are running upwards from sacrum to occiput. Gnawing hunger as the goneness in heart extends to the stomach. Pulse is arrhythmic and feeble but least disturbances may cause palpitation with weakness of heart. Moves continuously as she fears that if she stops moving the heart will stop beating and she will die. Sleeplessness. Post-diphtheric paralysis; dull aching pains in head are relieved by profuse urination. General ailments from heat of sun or hot summer.

She has nervous excitement. There is fear. Sensitive and nervous lady, very irritable - excited easily. Lack of courage. Fear of death but has no courage to die. Involuntary discharges from fright. Goes weak and exhausted due to excessive fear.

MODALITIES :

< Thinking of ailments, mental excitement, shock, 10 a.m. hot summer, damp weather.

> Continuous motion, profuse urination.

8.7.2 CIMICIFUGA

Non-progressive labour pains. Sensation as if she will pass stools during labour. False labour pains, much earlier than the expected date. Contraction of the uterus are non-rhythmic i.e. the progress of the labour is not coinciding with the pains. The pains are settled after passing stools. Spasmodic pain in the abdomen. The os is rigid. There is characteristic bearing down sensation. Pains in the ovarian region which travel upwards and downwards along the thighs. Ovarian neuralgia during pregnancy and during labour is well treated by this remedy. These pains move across the hips in the first stage of labour. Distressing and tearing pain in uterine region during parturition. Labour pains are severe. They are tedious, spasmodic, with fits or cramps in legs with much exertion. Lady is sleepless with uncomfortable nauseating feeling all the time. Complaints from taking cold.

Soreness, numbness and jerking of all the muscles. She is unable to walk properly as there is much trembling of the body due to loss of control over muscular system. Rheumatism of mainly muscles of neck and back with stiffness and lameness. Sense of constriction with stitching pains. Chorea of the muscles of rested part of body. So this makes her sleepless. Alternate diarrhoea and constipation. Paralytic weakness of the whole body. Mental state alternates with diarrhoea and rheumatism. Epileptic spasms in a hysterical woman.

Lady is very suspicious, anxious and restless. Fearful, fear of death with sadness. Sensation as if a black cloud has settled over her head. So everything seems to be dark and she becomes gloomy. Feels as if a heavy weight is on the head.

MODALITIES :

< Cold, motion, lying down.

> From warmth in general, eating.

8.7.3 COFFEA

Labour pains are ineffectual. There is ineffectual dilatation of cervical os. Contractions of uterus and extreme pressure on the os. There are false pains especially in the small of back. Intense and severe pains in the groins. During second stage, the characteristic bearing down pains need to be frequent and should be sustained. But in Coffea the pains are intermittent, therefore labour is delayed. Vulva and vagina are hypersensitive with voluptuous itching in the genital region. She has intolerance of tight clothing around abdomen. Severe but insufficient pains make her to cry as she is very sensitive to pains. Nervous excitement during labour. She sees visions and hears various noises. She does not like to be touched or even movements around her.

Neuralgic pains in the extremities which are more on exertion. The skin is dry; severe headache with sensation of tight bandage around the head, as if the brain would be torn to pieces, as if nail were driven into head. She has excessive hunger. Sleep is disturbed due to dreams.

Patient is very excited. She is full of ideas and has acute senses. Pleasurable impressions made her joyous. But sometimes she is very anxious and irritable. Easy comprehension of every matter and she is very alert and always ready to act.

MODALITIES :

< After excess of emotions, joy, strong odour, noise, open air, cold, night.

> warmth in general, on lying down.

8.7.4 ARSENICUM ALBUM

Contractions of the uterus are interrupted by painful sensitiveness of the uterus and the cervical os. There is great burning of vagina and vulva. Labour is weak and the uterus is flabby, therefore profuse bleeding after labour (PPH). This remedy is sometimes indicated in the last stage of labour when placenta remains adherent to uterus. Rigidity of the vagina and the uterus is weak so expulsion of foetal head is very difficult. Leucorrhoeal discharge before the onset of labour which excoriates the parts, causing itching and burning. Whitish thin discharge that burns the parts. Discharge is profuse and acrid. Cutting pain in lower part of abdomen which travel upwards.

Patient is prostrated and there is sinking of the vital state. It leads to frequent fainting attacks. Great burning pains with nervous prostration. Epileptic convulsions of the lady before or during the labour. Great dryness of mouth and she has to drink frequently to moisten her mouth. External burning pains with internal chill and the burning is ameliorated by warmth.

Mentally fear, anxiety and restlessness are marked features of Arsenic alb. lady. She is very fearful and has fear of death. Body is always covered with cold sweat. Hypersensitive and melancholic. Restlessness mentally due to fear and anxiety and suicidal thinking.

MODALITIES :

< Cold in general, right side. After mid-day, mid-night, cold food and drinks.

> Warmth in general, warm food and drinks, head elevation.

8.7.5 PULSATILLA

Uterine inertia with want of expulsive power causing retention of the foetus. Intermittent flow of blood. The uterine contractions are weak and feeble. They are also infrequent, thus labour becomes prolonged. She feels less pains, usually in the first stage and also in the second stage this trouble occurs. Foetal distress is likely to follow this hypotonic uterine inertia. Does not want abdomen to be covered. Prolapse of the bladder therefore incontinence of urine. Dyspnoea and palpitation during labour. She has chronic catarrh of genitalia and urethra. Copious mucous discharge through urogenital tract. Due to chronic catarrh and increased abdominal pressure there is increased frequency of micturition. Discharges from urogenital tract are thick, ropy, purulent or yellowish green and offensive. Deficient labour pains and spasmodic pains in abdomen and navel region make her unable to bear down. Plethoric patients. There is great exhaustion after labour. Exciting and fainting condition. Chilliness and pale face. It is said sometimes that Pulsatilla corrects malposition of the foetus by stimulating the muscular walls of the womb.

Pulsatilla lady is lean, thin and beautiful. She is very chilly but does not like to be covered and craves open air and is anyway aggravated from warm air. She always wants doors and windows open. Pains are of shooting and tearing type. They are always shifting. Discharges are also always changing. Patient's condition is worse from heat of bed and she is restless so cannot sleep until late night. Patient is having no thirst at all though her mouth is very dry. Chilliness and nausea are associated with the female complaints.

Mentally patient is very emotional and hypersensitive. She weeps easily. Fear of being alone and of darkness. Always changing mood. Tearful.

MODALITIES :

< Warm room, evening, left side, when feet hang down.

> Motion, cold drinks, open air, consolation.

8.7.6 CAULOPHYLLUM

After protracted and exhausting labour, reflex pains in back and chest. Spasmodic pains across lower abdomen. There is weakness in reproductive system of women. During parturition the contractions of uterus are too feeble to expel the contents. Many times they are only tormenting. Haematuria during labour. Relaxation of muscles and ligaments. There is heaviness in the lower abdomen. Sometimes prolapse of the uterus - subinvolution. Excoriating leucorrhoea. Os is extremely rigid and there are pains in the cervix as if pricks from needles. Severe spasmodic intermittent pains without any progress. Inharmonious contractions of the uterus. The uterine ligaments are over-stretched and thus relaxed. Spasmodic pains radiating from one site to another. Due to exhaustion patient is so prostrated that she cannot tolerate normal pains. She complains of profuse secretion from vagina. This remedy is well indicated in false pains.

Great weakness and exhaustion with lack of tonicity in muscular system. Rheumatic affections of small joints. Parts become very stiff. Pains are drawing and tearing. Pains fly from one site to another. Sense of fullness and tension in gastric region. Empty eructations with nausea and spasms of stomach due to uterine disturbances. Hysteria or choreic movements of various parts of body. Drooping of eyelid, especially upper eyelids. Pains are always paroxysmal.

MODALITIES :

< By taking stimulants like coffee and in open air.

> By releasing abdominal distension by passing flatus.

8.7.7 CINNAMONUM

There is bearing down sensation due to weak uterine supports. Ineffectual or false labour pains. She complains of spasmodic pain in the abdomen with twitching or fainting during labour. This remedy induces labour pains when there is complete cessation of labour pains. Severe metrorrhagia in primigravida after haemorrhage caused by overlifting during pregnancy. Profuse haemorrhage during puerperal period. The os is dilated but the placenta descends along with the head of foetus. Labour pains are increased so much that the lady is not able to tolerate them. Sleepy during labour. Post partum haemorrhage is bright red in colour.

Patient has no desire for anything. Haemorrhages from every natural orifice and mucous membrane. Epistaxis or metrorrhagia, haemoptysis and bleeding from intestines. Patient has gaseous distension of abdomen and may suffer from diarrhoea. Uterine bleeding may be due to strain at overlifting or by false step. Frequent, troublesome hiccough due to distension and uterine disturbances.

Other useful remedies for normal labour are

1) IPECACUANHA
2) PHOSPHORUS
3) CHAMOMILLA
4) IGNATIA
5) ARNICA

===========

TOPIC 8
POSTPARTUM HAEMORRHAGE

8.8.1 NITRIC ACID

Profuse uterine haemorrhage, when the third stage of labour is delayed. The placenta is very difficult to release and remains adherent to the uterus for a longer time. Nitric acid is known for profuse bleeding after long labour strain. Tachycardia, pallor and hypotension, these cardinal signs of shock are observed. The uterus is soft and flaccid. The blood is bright red or may be dark in colour. It is profuse and coagulable with stitching, piercing and lancinating pains in the region of uterus. There is violent pressure in the abdomen as if everything would come out. There is pain in small of back after haemorrhage. Pains radiate down the hips and thighs. There is weakness and nervous trembling of the body. Abdomen feels very sore with intense crampy pains. There is palpitation and neuralgic pain in every part. Itching and burning pains in genital region. Dyspnoea, shortness of breath. Every haemorrhage is attended with splinter-like pains. Pains are very violent, they come suddenly and go suddenly. Urine smells like horse's urine. Urine is dark brown in colour. Haemorrhage may cause sudden but ineffectual urging for stool. Stools are watery and acrid. Deafness from haemorrhage is better when she rides in a carriage.

She is very nervous, irritable and anxious. History of chronic disease behind this mental sphere. Tired, despondent and sad. Oversensitive to external impressions and great fear of death. Excitement causes nervous trembling.

MODALITIES :

< Extreme heat or cold, night.

> When moves passively.

8.8.2 PULSATILLA

The separation of the placenta is very difficult and it remains adherent to the uterus. If controlled corn traction is applied, then also it takes longer time to detach from the uterus. There is oozing of copious slow gushes of blood from the uterus.

There is heavy persistent pain in the uterus. Pressive pain in the abdomen and in the back. There is lameness of extremities as if the power is lost. There is ineffectual urge to pass stools. Pressing and drawing pains radiate towards the region of uterus. There is sense of constriction or constrictive pains in the left side of uterus. These pains make her to bend double. Blood flow is thick and changeable in character. There is changeability in flow. Blood flows, stops and flows again. Blood mixed with clots and watery flow. There is vomiting during blood flow.

Pulsatilla lady has her discharges and bleeding in profuse quantity. Burning in eyes with partial deafness. She is chilly patient and has nauseated feeling during haemorrhage. Complete absence of thirst. Offensive odour of mouth with great dryness. Feels smothered when she is lying down. Venous plethora with tearing and drawing pains in the joints. Neuralgic shooting pains. Oversensitiveness. She feels very uncomfortable and suffocated when in warm or closed room. She wants the doors and windows open. Overstraining may cause headache with stitching pains.

Mentally she is very emotional and has tearful mood. Fearful in the evening and in dark places or when she is alone. Consolation relieves her trouble and she desires sympathy from others. Cannot narrate her complaints without weeping.

MODALITIES:

< Rest, lying on left side, heat in general, evening.

> Sitting erect, open cold air, moving about or any motion.

8.8.3 CINCHONA OFFICINALIS

Cinchona lady has got haemorrhagic diathesis and she bleeds continuously and copiously. Blood is dark and clotted. The uterus is very atonic and causes profuse haemorrhage. Pallor or bluishness of the face and extremities. Tinnitus, vertigo and insensibility. Uterine colic leads to paroxysmal expulsion of blood and clots. Body becomes cold and cyanosed. She becomes greatly prostrated after the haemorrhage. Inflammation of the uterus which causes profuse haemorrhage. When China patient bleeds, there are cramps in muscles and convulsion sets in. During labour and after expulsion of the baby profuse uncoagulable haemorrhage is marked.

She bleeds and thus is much exhausted and she has no strength to do any physical work. Trembling of whole body. China causes anaemia and dropsies due to chronic haemorrhages. Even the perspiration causes great weakness and she has painless diarrhoea, worse in the night times. Due to haemorrhage she complains of sustained headache. Sensation as if the brain is striking on the skull surface. Dull headache. Headache is worse by touch, contact and mental exertion but she is better by moving. Vertigo and vomiting.

Despondent and tearful lady. Sleepless due to crowding of ideas and thoughts. Very disobedient and does not care for the feelings of others. Tossing about in bed and she has sudden burst of crying.

MODALITIES :

< Bending, draught of air, night, touch.

> Open air, hard pressure, warmth.

8.8.4. USTILAGO MAYDIS

Uterus is flaccid when it is felt per abdomen and there is painful burning condition in the ovarian region. Uterus may be hypertrophied but always atonic and unable to deliver the placenta. Pains are feeble. Dilated and relaxed os. Profuse salivation with burning sensation along the oesophagus and stomach. Blood is bright red or sometimes it is dark and clotted. Any motion or touch causes oozing of blood and the blood is drawn into long and dark strings. Profuse lochia. Palpitation with feeble pulse. Colicky pain in abdomen and painful contraction of the muscles of the extremities.

Uterus is hypertrophied and any stimulus may induce profuse haemorrhage. Palpitation. First tachycardia then feeble pulse. Sensation as if boiling water is flowing on the back. Dull and aching pains on the lumbar region. Dry skin and muscle cramp in the lower extremities.

Nervous lady with intense nymphomania. Mentally she is irritable and depressed. Despondent.

MODALITIES :

< Any touch or motion.

> At rest.

8.8.5 CINNAMONUM

The Cinnamonum lady is weak and debilitated, feeble and anaemic due to history of haemorrhages like menorrhagia or malaena. There is relaxation of the smooth muscles in the body and this leads to relaxation of the vessels especially arteries leading to copious, bright red blood flow. Any strain on the muslces of loin brings out fresh red haemorrhage from the uterus. She has intense bearing down pains with plethora. Haemorrhage may appear some days after the delivery. Blood is clear and not mixed with clots.

Cinnamonum lady is chlorotic or anaemic. She presents with the history of chronic metrorrhagia or menorrhagia. Haemorrhage when she missteps while walking or makes any physical exertion.

MODALITIES :

< Physical exertion, any strain.

> At rest.

8.8.6 NUX VOMICA

Blood from the uterus is black. There may be uterine inertia. She faints frequently due to bleeding. She feels as if the bowels wanted to move. The postpartum haemorrhage of Nux vomica is always associated with the complaint of constipation. She has uterine cramps and intense bearing down pains. Sacral pains are assoicated with constant urging to stool. Frequent desire for urination. Mental symptoms during this condition are very peculiar and useful to prescribe the remedy. She is very excitable, oversensitive and hyperimpressionable.

Severe backache and paralytic feeling in the extremities. Burning, bruised and neuralgic pains in the back. Cramps in legs. She is very chilly; she likes to be covered and the windows and doors to be closed. She is worse in a cold room. Convulsions set in due to any external stimulus and she is conscious at the time of convulsions. History of alternate diarrhoea and constipation. Though there is frequent urging, the stools or urine are passed only in small quantity in each effort or sitting.

Mentally Nux vomica lady is sensitive and emotional. Becomes angry very easily. Anxious and impatient. Low muttering delirum. Nervous lady. She wants to be alone.

MODALITIES :

< Mental or physical strain, dry and cold air.

> Damp wet weather, at rest, lying down.

8.8.7 TRILLIUM PENDULUM

Trillium is having haemorrhage from any orifice. All the pelvic organs are relaxed. The blood is bright red in colour. She feels as if the hips and thighs would break to pieces. Veins feel as if they are loaded and the parts feel too tight. If she has chronic haemorrhage, then later on she may become anaemic and the character of blood changes to pale. She has faintness and dizziness during the haemorrhage. Bearing down pains. Urine dribbles, after parturition.

She has chronic bleeding complaints, making her anaemic. Bleeding from nose, mouth, lungs, bowels etc. There are cramp-like pains everywhere. Fullness of vessels are also well marked. Headache with blurring of vision. Passes pure blood per rectum instead of stools. Haemorrhage brings on great prostration to her. Her limbs are cold and there is tachycardia. Dyspnoea with shooting pains in the chest. Patient is forgetful and confused. She is anxious and gets disturbed easily by any noise.

MODALITIES :

< Exertion.

> Tight bandage around hips.

Other useful remedies for postpartum haemorrhage are

1) MILLEFOLIUM
2) IPECACUANHA
3) ACETIC ACID
4) HAMAMELIS VIRGINICA
5) SECALE CORNUTUM

============

TOPIC 9

PUERPERAL PSYCHOSIS

8.9.1 STRAMONIUM

Puerperal convulsions are well treated by this remedy. Patient complains of anxiety and convulsions since first trimester. Puerperal convulsions have septic nature. She thinks that she has committed many mistakes and she has to die but she is still alive. Convulsions precipitated during pregnancy or during labour. She has poor sleep and shortness of breath. She has sense of constriction or sense of pressure on the chest, thus cannot breath freely. Nymphomania with obscene language is marked. Face is red, eyes are flushed. Incoherent speech. Cerebral congestion with delirium. Stertorous breathing. Mouth is open as lower jaw is paralyzed. During convulsions, due to injury to tongue bloody discharges from mouth. Violent headache. Irritation of brain from constant dwelling upon a subject.

8.9.2 VERATRUM ALBUM

This lady is very violent and excited, throughout the pregnancy and also when goes into labour. She has destructive tendency. Tears her cloths, goes on praying in loud voice. She has mania with desire to cut. She has violent, religious and lascivious mania too. Each attack is with a single mania at a time. Sadness and melancholia. Hopelessness and she sits in a corner and broods. She may become lascivious and has kissing mania or nymphomania. Excitation and exhaustion of the nerve powers. Impending misfortunes.

Indifferent to everything. Stupor, she sits like stupid person and has no intention to observe anything.

8.9.3 PLATINA

Hysterical condition of both mind and body. General hyperaesthesia. She thinks that everything is changed and she feels that everybody around her has committed some mistakes. She has strong impulses to kill the baby and she is weary of everything.

8.9.4 BELLADONNA

A woman in confinement shows various signs of hyperaesthesia. Oversensitive to noise, sound and even the breeze of air. Wants to close the windows to prevent the air entery into the room. Does not want touch of the bed to her body. Little jar aggravates the conditions. These symptoms are usually observed after 2-3 days. Very quarrelsome, goes on spitting or biting. All these are following difficult or painful labour. Violent convulsions are marked, associated with cerebral congestion. Motion increases the action of heart and she complains of palpitation but no throbbing. Violence is marked which is said to be active and never passive. She is in wild state, striking, tearing, biting the things and doing all meaningless things. She is in a state of excitability. She is full of imaginations. The puerperal fever may predipose this condition.

8.9.5 CICUTA VIROSA

Nervous system is affected in puerperal Psychosis. There is increased irritability due to pressure on the genital tract during labour. Pressure and the progress of labour cause convulsions. Everything seems to be strange and terrible. If the convulsion sets in, it extends from centre to circumference. Vertigo with gastralgia. There is violent muscular spasm. Sudden and violent shocks from head to other parts of the body. Does not like to take food or to be nourished. The gastric symptom starts prior to any nervous dysfunction. Nausea and gastritis give the alarming signals as the trouble would start any moment, patient herself can feel when the trouble would start. Heaviness of the head. There is sensation of coldness in the extremities. The whole body is tense. Unable to recognise family members. Fails to recollect what has occurred just few minutes before. She is melancholic and indifferent. Strange and vivid dreams. Touch and little noise bring on convulsions. Irrelevent talk confused state of mind. Does not remember the past or what has occurred during that period. Difficult hearing.

8.9.6 AGNUS CASTUS

This remedy is usually indicated for the nursing patients. The milk ceases after she has started feeding or the quantity reduces. Thus the lady becomes sad and anxious. Uterine haemorhage associated with puerperal psychosis. Severe pain in abdomen with derangement of the mind. Fetid leucorrhoea. There is great irritability of mind with pricking and tingling sensation everywhere in the body. Patient is disgusted due to the disease. She is pitiful. She has loss of memory. Despair and suicidal thoughts. She is anxious about her baby and its growth. Worried about her condition, goes on thinking as how these sequences of events have occurred in her life. Desperate about the things. Hopeless condition of mind. Cannot concentrate her mind, she looks puzzled. Tearing pains in the muscles of neck and face. She is anaemic with lymphadenitis.

8.9.7 CIMICIFUGA

Puerperal psychosis is due to high grade fever, after second or third day of puerperium with anxiousness, restlessness and full of tears calls for this remedy. She has fear of death with excitement. Great suspicion of the mind. Even when given a medicine, she will refuse it, thinking that there may be something wrong about it. Puerperal mania from taking cold during or soon after labour. She is melancholic, gloomy and low-spirited. Mental state is deteriorated. Severe pain in back during and after labour.

Pain in the uterine region, darting in nature, goes from side to side. Bearing down and pressive pains. The parts are relaxed and intermittent bleeding sets in. The flow generally relieves the pain. Some bruised feeling all over the head. Giddiness and loss of appetite. Bruised sensation in the occiput and on top of the head. There is sensation as if the top of head will fly off. This headache is better by being in cold air. Hysterical condition with pain in nape of neck. Many of these symptoms start in the pregnancy, aggravated during and after labour. Shivering in the first stage of labour. Hysterical condition with trembling of legs. Cannot walk easily. Numbness is such as if parts are paralyzed. Paralytic weakness of the muscles of the lower extremities.

Other important remedies for puerperal psychosis are

1. AGARICUS MUS.
2. ARUM TRIPHYLLUM
3. CANNABIS INDICA
4. HYOSCYAMUS
5. OPIUM

==============

TOPIC 10

PUERPERAL FEVER

8.10.1 TEREBINTHINA

Fever two days after parturition. Heat with violent thirst. Dry, brown tongue. There is profuse cold and clammy sweat. Stupor with delirium. There is bearing down sensation in the uterine region. Intense burning in epigastric and also in the right hypochondriac region. Bleeding from the uterus like dirty mud. Urine is cloudy and dark. Distension of abdomen. Nausea with vomiting. Headache with thirst. Pulse is thready and fast. Great prostration due to heavy perspiration. Parts are inflamed and red hot.

Feels drowsy all the time and has dull headache with tired feeling. Tympanic distension of abdomen with melaena. Constant tenesmus and strangury. Burning pains in abdomen, especially in kidney and uterine region. Various types of skin eruptions. Puerperal peritonitis is the cause of fever. Neuralgic pains in the sensory organs. Tinnitus. Feels prostrated and goes in stuporous condition.

8.10.2 KREOSOTUM

Stitching pain in the vagina with inflammatory condition of the mucous membrane. High degree of fever due to urogenital tract infection. Infection spreads from vagina to uterus. But pains travel from umbilical region to vagina. Very offensive, putrid and excoriating lochia, persisting almost all the time, ceases for very short time. Offensive urine with cloudy, brown appearance. There is violent itching of vulva and vagina. Excessive vaginal secretions—yellow, acrid with odour of green corn. Itching worse towards evening. Burning in soles with high degree of fever. She has bleeding tendency. Small wounds bleed profusely. Lips are red. Dull pain in the frontal and occipital regions during fever. During fever stage she becomes very violent and irritable. Hot and red face is expressive of the sufferings. Haemorrhages, puffiness, ulcers and gangrene formation is also seen in case of puerperal derangements. Sudden and uncontrollable urge to urinate. Cough with free expectoration. Hoarseness of voice associated with laryngeal pains. Paralytic feeling. Intense itching with burning. Arthralgia. Distension of abdomen.

Peevish, stupid lady with vanishing of thoughts. Forgetful. Dull headache. Irritable and despondent. Weeps easily and music causes weeping and palpitation.

MODALITIES :

< Rest, lying in bed, cold open air.

> Warmth in general, motion.

8.10.3 PULSATILLA

Itching and burning in the eyes with high degree of fever. Genital parts are sensitive due to inflammation. There is sense of continuous pressure on the uterus. Tendency to stupor. Catarrh with acute cold and fever. Dry tongue yet refuses water. Patient is thirstless. Pain in joints after parturition. Dyspepsia with great tightness of abdomen after meals. Coryza with stoppage of right nostril. There are pressing type of pains at the root of nose. Wandering, stitching pains in head. These pains extend to face and settle in teeth. Thick bland discharge from nose and eyes. Affections of upper respiratory tract. Hoarseness of voice appears and disappears. Soreness in chest and in nipples. Urine emitted with cough. Cough is associated with expectoration which is bland, thick, bitter and greenish. Shooting pains in back and in between the shoulder blades. During febrile condition there are drawing tensive pains in thighs and legs with restlessness, sleeplessness and chilliness. Chill even in warm room. External heat is intolerable; veins are distended. During pyrexia she complains of headache, nausea, diarrhoea and loss of appetite.

Pulsatilla has great intolerance of warmth or heat so she craves for open and fresh air. The mental and physical spheres during fever is ever changing. Sleep is disturbed. Feels as if the limbs are paralysed. Breath is very offensive with bitter taste in mouth. History of amenorrhoea from getting the feet wet. Tearing pains everywhere in the body. Eruptive fevers and urticaria. Involuntary urination and diarrhoea. Limbs are red, hot and inflamed with feeling of soreness.

She is very sensitive and timid. Weeps easily. Easily discouraged. Likes sympathy from others.

MODALITIES :

< Warmth in general, evening.

> Open and fresh air.

8.10.4 SECALE CORNUTUM

She has every tendency to putrescence. There is bloody, copius discharge with tingling sensation in extremities. Great prostration. Skin is shrivelled and dusky blue in appearance. Varicose ulcers are well marked. As this lady has got tendency to habitual abortion in third month, she is prone to get uro-genital infections. Even in febrile condition the parts are cold and dry. Clammy sweat with excessive thirst. Though the fever cannot be felt from outside, she has internal feeling of heat. She has great aversion to heat in any form. Formication under skin. Burning sensation in any part is better by cold and wants parts uncovered though they are cold to touch. Suppression or retention of urine. Painless prolonged bearing down sensation. Offensive diarrhoea during fever. Pulse is feeble, rapid respiration, difficult breathing. Burning fever interrupted by shaking chills, cold limbs, cold sweat over whole body calls for this remedy.

MODALITIES :

< Heat in general, covering.

> Cold in general, open air, massage and uncovering the parts.

8.10.5 BELLADONNA

Puerperal fever particularly after suppression of the milk. Also due to puerperal peritonitis. Onset is violent as if hot steam is issuing from the body. Great distension and sensitiveness of the abdomen after delivery. Retention of urine, passes drop by drop. Involuntary urination and stools during febrile condition. Stitching and digging pains coming suddenly and disappearing suddenly. Violent spasmodic pains in extremities as if the parts were grasped in claws. Restless sleep, cries out due to pains. Sleeplessness with drowsiness. High fever but relatively low toxaemia. Burning, and steaming heat. Feet are icy cold. Peripheral circulation is increased and skin becomes dry, red and hot. Profuse perspiration, more on the head. No thirst in heat stage.

Belladonna is known for violence of the symptoms. Sudden onset of fever and rises to its peak within short time. Face is red and hot, flushed. Skin is also dry, red, shining and intolerably hot. Pupils are dilated. Retention of urine or oliguria. She has no thirst during heat stage but feels little thirsty during chill stage. Only upper parts are congested so feels hot. Lower limbs are icy cold. Barking cough with chest pain. Cramps in stomach.

She becomes violent and maniacal during fever. Offends, strikes and bites everybody. Furious state of mind. Hallucinations, delirium.

MODALITIES :

< Lying down, draught of air, touch.

> Sitting in semi-erect position.

8.10.6 AILANTHUS GLANDULOSA

High degree of fever with throat infection followed by parturition. Tonsillar glands are oedematous, dusky red with difficulty in swallowing. There is much swelling of tonsillar glands both external and internal. Dry cough with choking sensation. Ichorous and fetid leucorrhoea. There is delirium during high fever. Miliary livid rash on the skin. Large blisters filled with dark coloured fluid. Constant thirst during febrile stage. Intense irritability during fever with soreness, pricking and tingling sensation everywhere in the body.

During fever she may suffer from diarrhoea or dysentery. Dusky face, tongue is very dry and brown. Dry cough with tired feeling in lungs. Hyperventilation. Hoarseness of voice with swelling of neck. Neck region is tender to touch. Intense photophobia. Passive congestion of head. Pupils are dilated.

8.10.7 LACHESIS

Puerperal fever with great loquacity. Lochia is fetid, urine is suppressed. Abdomen is distended, cannot bear the least pressure of clothings. Sore throat. Inflammation of the tonsillar glands, worse on left side. She can swallow solids but liquids are more painful to swallow. Parotid glands are inflamed. Tonsils are purplish in colour. There is sense of something solid in throat and wants to swallow. There is sensation of pain in chest region radiating from uterus. Skin is alternately burning hot and icy cold.

There are flushes of heat and perspiration is also hot. Chill is felt mainly in the back. Venous congestion and haemorrhages. Skin bluish or purple. Oedematous affection of tonsils. She is constipated due to piles or pains in the rectum. Irregular pulse with tachycardia and she may become cyanosed during fever.

Suspicious lady. Talkative. Always restless and feels no comfort at all. She does not like to mix with anybody. Religious insanity. Dreams of fire and dead persons every second night.

MODALITIES :

< Pressure, heat in general, sleep.

> Warm applications and discharges.

Other important remedies for puerperal fever are

1. VERATRUM VIRIDE
2. OPIUM
3. CIMICIFUGA
4. CHAMOMILLA
5. ACONITUM NAPELLUS

****

TOPIC 11
RETAINED PLACENTA

8.11.1 CAULOPHYLLUM

This is one of the leading remedies in retained placenta, complication of third stage of labour. It is prolonged beyond half an hour. This prolongation of expulsion of the placenta from the uterus is mainly due to three causes. First one is the feeble contractions of the uterus. They are too feeble to expel the placenta out and it remains adherent to uterus. Second reason is the weakness of supports of uterus and weakness of the reproductive system as a whole. Third cause is the uterine inertia. Relaxation of muscles of uterus causes prolapse and sense of heaviness. Profuse bleeding. Needle-like pains in the cervix. Severe drawing, eractic pains in the region of uterus.

Haemorrhage of Caulophyllum is always of passive type and is due to the atonic or relaxed blood vessels. Blood goes on oozing sometimes for hours together. Congested uterus may cause acrid leucorrhoea which causes much prostration. Drawing and tearing pain in legs. Back and neck muscles are stiff and lame. Very much hysterical, irritable, apprehensive and restless lady. Sleepless; sensitive to cold; likes warmth.

8.11.2 BELLADONNA

Belladonna patient has the tendency to get recurrent attacks of infections. These infections result in inflammation of the parts. Acute inflammation of the uterus with enlargement of the uterus. Bearing down sensation. There are morbid adhesions due to these recurrent infections. Uterus is congested and is relaxed, tired, weak and stretched. It is suited to the women who are extremely sensitive and plethoric. Retained placenta in women who have married late in life and have become pregnant. There is history of threatened abortion. During delivery the muscle fibres of uterus are in a state of tension. Uterus will not relax. Hour glass constriction. The flow of blood is fresh, dark red and hot. Blood gushes from the vagina. Great induration of the parts. Tenderness of abdominal wall.

Everywhere in the body there is great dryness and heat. Congestion is also widely seen. Spasmodic affections of hollow organs and it leads to severe colicky pain and other disturbances. Parts are swollen due to congestion and there is throbbing pain. Affected parts are very sensitive to touch, jar, motion etc. Any external stimulus may induce convulsions. The parts are very much hot, cannot touch those. Change of position brings on vertigo and she feels as if she is falling backwards. Pain in ileo-caecal region and that area becomes painful to touch. Heat and pains around umbilical region and there is sense of constriction.

Active and violent mental symptoms. She becomes wild, bites, strikes and tears things. Furious rage and anger. She uses absurd language and she has fear of imaginary things. Hallucination, illusion, and delusion. Aversion to light, company, noise etc. She feels better in dark. Anxiety and excitement with palpitation. Hyperaesthesia.

MODALITIES :

< Draught of air, touch, jar, motion, any smell.

> In dark and warm room, rest, semi-erect posture.

8.11.3 CANTHARIS

Rapid settlement of inflammation in the uterine region. She is hypersensitive. All the parts are inflamed and tender to touch. Inflammation of uterine wall and ovaries. There is intense burning in the vagina. The normal contracting power of the uterus is lost. No explusive pains are present. Therefore placenta is retained. Puerperal convulsions after retained placenta. Violent lancinating pains through kidneys and back. Passes stools at the time of urination. Retention of urine with cutting pains. Tenesmus after parturition. Urinary organs and genitalia are in a state of inflammation. Retained placenta in Cantharis has a history of gonorrhoea. Violent inflammation with high intensity of burning and rapidity of pains are the indications of this remedy.

Violent inflammation of the whole system and there is intense burning of the parts. Violent congestive headache and she feels as if stabbed with knife. Retention of urine, strangury. Violent lancinating pains in back. She has oversensitiveness of all parts and intense burning in the vagina, ameliorated by rubbing it. Scalding and smarting pain at the last drop of urine and she cries. Profound prostration and hippocratic look of the face. She is very much thirsty but has fear of drinking water as it aggravates her condition. There is constant and uncontrollable urging to urinate.

Hot head, red face with excitement and delirium and she may become unconscious. Great confusion. Nymphomania. Delirium; talks about sex and related things. Fear of water.

MODALITIES :

< Cold water, touch, urination.

> Rubbing the parts.

8.11.4 SECALE CORNUTUM

This remedy produces ulcers on the endometrium. These ulcers form background for the morbid adhesions of the placenta. Therefore uterine contractions are not uniform. Ulcerations with sloughs retain the placenta. Discharge of black coloured blood, liquid in nature, lasts for longer time. There is offensive, venous bleeding from the uterus. Vaginal discharges are offensive. Violent inflammation of uterus, ovaries and cervical canal. Expulsion of blood clots with severe stinging, neuralgic pain in uterine region. Convulsions of the parts with cramps in calf muscles and thighs.

Mentally the lady is very nervous and anxious. Stupor. Weak memory. Fear of death is also marked and her face becomes anaemic and expressive of fear. She has tendency to behave like a mad and she may become impulsive.

MODALITIES :

< Heat in general, touch, covering.

> Cold application, open air, uncovering, rubbing.

8.11.5 PULSATILLA

There is venous congestion of uterine region. Veins are engorged and there is venous stasis. Thus there is rise in temperature of uterus. This fullness and redness hamper the uterine contractions. Therefore it is very difficult for placenta to get detached from uterus. Profuse bleeding from venous congestion. There is intense burning of uterus and cervial os. Blanc discharges with profuse haemorrhage. Distension of abdomen with oversensitiveness. Chronic constipation. Frequent urination during parturition. But quantity is less. Involuntary urination while coughing and sneezing. Severe pain in abdomen makes her to bend double. When Pulsatilla lady is taken to the labour room, she always wants the windows and doors open as she has great longing for open and cold air. Abdomen is sensitive to touch. All the discharges are greenish-yellow and bland. Only the leucorrhoea is acrid and milky. There is all-gone sensation in stomach and pelvis. Burning pains in palms and soles. Tongue is also burning and dry but then also there is no thirst. Changeability is well marked in Pulsatilla lady. Spasmodic, colicky pain in the uterine region. Tearing, jerking pain in the extremities and she is restless due to these shifting pains. Burning pains and haematuria. Bladder is irritated and she cannot hold the urine. Involuntary urination when intra-abdominal pressure is raised.

Mentally she is very gentle and has yielding disposition. Dull mood. Weeps easily. Fear of ghosts. Consolation ameliorates her immediately.

MODALITIES :

< Warmth in general, evening, lying on left side.

> Cold in general, sitting erect, pressure, motion, open air.

8.11.6 SABINA

Sabina lady has haemorrhagic diathesis. She is having early menarche and history of abortion, especially at third month. There is great atony of uterus so labour is premature. This leads to the condition like retained placenta. Pains are paroxysmal and there occurs uterine colic due to the retained placenta. After-pains are very intolerable. There are drawing pains from sacrum to pubis and she feels as if the bones of pelvis are separated. Pains are from below upwards too. Copious haemorrhage, the blood is partly clotted and partly fluid; active haemorrhage. Prostration and anaemia. Worse in warm room. Music is intolerable.

Sabina lady is having past history of gonorrhoea and the sycotic miasm is predominant in background. She may also give history of rheumatism. She is very hot and has violent pulsations everywhere in body. Burning pains in the region of kidney with haematuria. She has bearing down pains in abdomen with sense of constriction. Intense lancinating pains from pit of stomach to back. History of menorrhagia, metrorrhagia. Skin is showing outgrowths with burning and itching. Gouty nodosities. Pains shoot up from vagina to uterus or sometimes umbilicus too.

Music is unbearable for Sabina patient and it makes her nervous. She feels as if the music passes through her bones and marrow.

MODALITIES :

< Warm room, heat in general, motion, any change of position, haemorrhage.

> Open air, cold, fresh air.

8.11.7 IPECACUANHA

Ipecac lady is also having haemorrhagic diathesis, but the miasm is psora in the background of her complaints. Her symptoms are always attended with nausea and vomiting. Labour pains are very poor and the uterus is not contracting properly. Profuse bright red arterial haemorrhage which gushes out. Sharp pinching pain in the umbilical region moves down to the uterus. Every flow makes her to gasp and she has feeling of fainting. Haemorrhage causes great pallor, exhaustion and sometimes syncope also. Bleeding from relaxed uterus. Constant nausea and vomiting.

History of epistaxis or bleeding from intestine, haematuria, haematemesis etc. When she sees any moving object it nauseates her. Shortness of breath with sense of constriction in chest. Exertion causes haemoptysis. Her body is stretched and the limbs are jerking and come towards each other. Tongue is clean and there is profuse salivation but complete absence of thirst. Perspiration of only upper part of body, it is sour smelling. She has cold sweat on forehead.

MODALITIES :

< Dry, warm air, any movement, lying down.

Other useful remedies for retained placenta are

1) SEPIA
2) ARSENICUM ALBUM
3) CIMICIFUGA
4) GOSSYPIUM
5) ARNICA MONTANA

==============

TOPIC 12

RETENTION OF URINE AFTER LABOUR

8.12.1 ARNICA MONTANA

Retention of urine due to prolonged labour. Third stage of the labour is prolonged. Due to this, the overstretching of bladder muscle takes place. Fibres of bladder are injured. This blunt trauma by head of foetus indicates Arnica. Retention of urine with great urge to pass the urine. Urine is dark coloured and offensive in nature. Acidic in character. This causes intense burning and irritation to the bladder. Therefore there is also increased frequency of micturition. Urethra is sore. There is bruised feeling from bladder neck to urethra. The urine is brown or inky with piercing pain in the bladder as from a knife plunged into the kidney.

Along with retention of urine she may suffer from involuntary offensive diarrhoea. Sore, lame, bruised feeling all over the body and she feels as if she is beaten by something. Due to intolerable pains, she cannot lie on any surface and feels it very hard. Head is hot and rest of the body is cold. Injury results in soreness of nipples and bruised feeling in the private parts.

8.12.2 CAUSTICUM

This remedy has two-fold action on a patient who complains of retention of urine after parturition. One is on paralysis of bladder due to overstretching. The muscles of the bladder are overstretched during parturition and lose their tonicity or sometimes the centre in the brain is affected which controls the action of the bladder. Muscles of the bladder get paralysed and lose their function to evacuate the contents of the bladder. Involuntary dribbling of urine while standing and lying down. She expels very little quantity of urine and very slowly. Sometimes stops voiding urine. Retention from slightest excitement and after parturition or surgical operation. She complains of losing the sense in urethra. Progressive paralysis of every system and every organ. The parts feel very much burning with rawness and soreness. Dry heat in the body with uterine inertia. Drowsy in daytime but cannot sleep at night due to worries or some chronic ailments. Restless.

Sad, hopeless and cries easily. She has history of long-standing grief. Sympathetic to every person.

MODALITIES :

< Clear fine weather, cold in general.

> Heat in general, damp wet weather.

8.12.3 HYOSCYAMUS

Due to long-lasting labour pains Hyoscyamus patient has retention of urine. Twitching of the muscles of bladder takes place and there are severe pains from baldder to coccyx. Violent burning urine. Passes little quantity and involuntarily. She has kind of delirium where she passes urine after hearing the noise of water. She becomes violent after retention of urine. Typical spasmodic pains in the urinary bladder. Inflammation of the trigon of the bladder. She has no will for urination.

Sleeplessness and restlessness due to muscular pains and dilated pupils. Vomiting relieves her pains. Sense of intoxication. Distension of abdomen with colicky pains. Convulsions in general.

Nymphomania, in jealous and confused lady. Deep comatose state, very talkative and suspicious. Irresistible desire to laugh at everything.

MODALITIES :

< Lying down, at night, after food.

> Stooping or bending forward.

8.12.4 NUX VOMICA

Nux vomica lady has irritable bladder due to traumatic injury at the time of labour. The sphincter of urinary bladder is not functioning properly, therefore there is involuntary micturition. Patient strains but the sphincter is paralysed so fails to pass the urine. Neuralgic pains in the baldder. There is sense of pulling or tension in the walls of bladder. Drawing pains in the sacrum and hips. Paralytic condition of the bladder due to over-stimulation. Cutting and colicky pains while urinating. Pain shoots to the rectum and she has urge for stool. Increased frequency of micturition. Haematuria. Itching in the urethra while urinating.

Along with the retention of urine the lady may complain of constipation and there is frequent but ineffectual desire to pass the stool. Feels uneasy in the rectum. Dyspepsia with nausea and vomiting. Irritation of all the organs. Dribbling of urine causes pruritus vulvae. Paralytic feeling in the extremities. Patient feels chilly all the time. More chill when she is uncovered but she does not like to be uncovered. Burning and hot sensations all over the skin.

Nux vomica lady is always spiteful and irritable. She can not bear any mistakes and scolds everybody. She has feeling that time passes too slowly. She does not like to be touched.

MODALITIES :

< When uncovered, touch, dry weather.

> Pressure, damp wet weather.

8.12.5 CANTHARIS

Cutting pains with tenesmus. She has desire for stool while urinating. During labour she feels if she could pass little urine, she will be better. She strains for voiding the urine, but she does not succeed. Thus there is no relief of the symptom. All the parts of urinary tract are inflamed and sensation as if they are on fire. She has tenesmus not only when bladder is full but also when it is empty. Retention of urine due to trauma from head of foetus. Due to this trauma there is irritation. Violent pains with frequent urging for urination. Urine is bloody and burns as if there is fire in the bladder. Suppression of urine after parturition. The intensity, the rapidity, the burning and the typical anxiety of the patient indicates Cantharis.

Cantharis is also useful in the puerperal convulsions. Her face is pale and wretched. She has intense burning everywhere and this burning is better only by cold applications and rubbing forcefully. Every touch produces spasm or contraction of the part. Palms and soles are very cold with cold sweat. Tearing and lancinating pains in the coccygeal region.

She has great restlessness and furious delirium. May become unconscious suddenly. Cries due to the troubles. There may be nymphomania during puerperium.

MODALITIES :

< From taking coffee, touch, while urinating.

> Rubbing the parts, cold application.

8.12.6 EQUISETUM

Severe dull pains in the bladder region with sensation as if the bladder is full. This fulness of bladder is not at all relieved by passing urine. After she goes into labour, she has frequent desire to pass urine even though there are severe pains at the tip of urethra at the time of urination. Passes very little quantity of urine at a time and that too drop by drop. There are sharp burning and cutting pains in urethra while urinating. Incontinence of urine after labour. She has history of retention and dysuria during pregnancy and the same symptoms may relapse after delivery. Urine is turbid with albuminuria.

Mainly right sided affections. Passes albumin in the urine. Tenderness of the right lumbar region. Painful urination. Loss of control over bladder and bowels. She has more pains when she lies on right side and it also causes dribbling of urine. Worse at night and there are fearful dreams.

MODALITIES :

< Touch, pressure, lying on right side, night.

> By lying down.

8.12.7 GELSEMIUM

Retention of urine due to nervous excitement and shock. General suppression of urine when patient goes to labour. In fact she passes profuse, clear watery urine but when she goes into labour, quantity is decreased. Urine is retained due to paralytic condition of the sphincter. Many times she is febrile and in this condition she loses control over the bladder and passes urine involuntarily. Confused state of mind, therefore continuous dribbing of urine. Cannot control the flow, paralytic weakness of the musles of bladder. Congestive state of the sphincter. There are drawing, cramping pains from bladder to back and then under left shoulder blade. Intermitent flow due to muscular weakness, muscles of the back feel bruised during labour with retention of urine.

The troubles in Gelsemium lady are due to the weakness and paralytic changes in the muscular system. Dullness and drowsiness are the associated complaints of the patient in every ailment. There is trembling of the body due to loss of control over the muscles. Respiration is very slow and she has sense of weariness and tiredness in the chest. Disturbed sleep or loss of sleep. Dull, heavy pains with easy fatiguability.

Delirium in sleep. She feels dizzy and prostrated. Paralysis due to mental derangement.

MODALITIES :

< Excitement, damp weather.

> Passing the urine, motion, open air, bending forward.

Other important remedies for retention of urine after labour are

1) BELLADONNA
2) ARSENICUM ALBUM
3) OPIUM
4) LYCOPODIUM
5) RHUS TOXICODENDRON

===========

TOPIC 13
STERILITY

8.13.1 NATURM MURIATICUM

Nat. mur is the indicated remedy for sterility where the uterus is intensely sore. Inflammation of the endometrium. Useful in infertility due to vaginal factors such as vaginismus and vaginitis. Patient complains of leucorrhoea which is acrid and whitish in nature. When secondary infection sets in leucorrhoea turns yellowish and then green. She has the tendency to take cold. Even the breath of cold air makes her sick. The vagina is very sensitive, and is dry. There is sensation as if numerous pins are pricking in the vagina. Complete vaginal mucosa is dry producing dyspareunia.

Nat mur. lady has got debilitating conditions like anaemia or leucocytosis. She is feeling tired all the time. Feeling of weariness. Known cases of diabetes mellitus. Marked emaciation, more in the neck. Dropsical condition and oedema everywhere due to sodium retention. Palpitation and arrhythmic pulse. Irregular menses or amenorrhoea. She feels very hot during menses.

There may be a mental cause in the background of diseases. History of suppressed grief, fear or desires. She feels very awkward and so behaves hastily. Easily excitable. She may be hysterical. Weeps after laughing. Desires to be alone and cries due to suppressed emotions.

MODALITIES :

< Mental worries, heat, conversation, music, noise.

> Open cold air, tight clothing.

8.13.2 PHOSPHORICUM ACIDUM

It is a great remedy for primary sterility due to debilitated conditions such as tuberculosis, diabetes mellitus. It also acts well in the patients who grow rapidly. Obesity is well marked. Due to hypothalamic dysfunction she develops diabetes which results in defective ovulation. Therefore menses are too profuse and too early. Irregular menses make fertilisation very difficult. Due to debility resistence is lowered. So she is exposed to.a variety of infections, systemic as well as local. There is profuse leucorrhoea which is acrid and yellowish and caüses irritation of the parts. The pH of the vaginal secretions turn into acidic form, therefore the sperms which are deposited there die soon. There is inflammation of the endometrium causing the parts to be sore and tender. General signs of septic condition.

Lips and tongue are dry and cracked so she has intense craving for juicy or refreshing things. Abdomen is distended. Chronic dyspepsia. History of early menarche. Grief causes palpitation and other physical ailments. Chronic diarrhoea makes the lady debilitated and rachitic. Earthy and anaemic look of face. Deafness or tinnitus in ears. Alopecia or early greying of the hair in young patient. Blue rings around the eyes. Photophobia. Dyspnoea and weakness in chest. Beating and boring pains in back in beween the scapulae. Copious perspiration.

Lady becomes indifferent and apathetic. Forgetful due to weak memory. She cannot find correct meaningful word for any conversation. Also she cannot understand any speech or any matter. All this is due to grief or shock. Delirious condition of mind.

MODALITIES :

< Conversation, sexual excess.

> When remains warm.

8.13.3 BORAX

Borax patient has peculiar leucorrhoea probably due to secondary monilial infection. Leucorrhoea is like white of an egg with sensation as if warm water was flowing through the genitals. She has membranous dysmenorrhoea. Endometrial layer continuously sheds off. So no bed for fertilised ovum. This naturally results in difficult conception. There are labour-like pains during menses. There is infection of genitals producing eczema of the genitalia. This patient also complains of pruritus vulvae.

Borax has irritation of each and every system in the body. Great heat everywhere in the body. Eruptions and wrinkled skin. Every swelling is red and shiny. Psoric complaints. Distension of the distal parts. Pains with eructations. Trembling of the whole body. Tangled or split hair. Aching violent. Disturbed sleep with voluptuous dreams. History of membranous dysmenorrhoea.

Nervousness is marked. Frightful and anxious. Extreme fear of thunderstorm.

MODALITIES :

< Polluted air; dust; warm weather.

8.13.4 PLATINA

Platina lady has intense vaginismus with chronic cervicitis. She is prone to get recurrent urogenital infections resulting in oophoritis, salpingitis and endometritis. Due to recurrent ovarian infections process of ovulation is hampered resulting in sterility. Increased sexual excitement and voluptuous crawling in the genitals. This is well recognised not as an inflammatory process, but as hyperaesthesia. There is itching and tingling in the external genital parts. Dryness of the parts with hyperaesthesia, therefore coition is painful. She is unable to complete the act. The vulva and vagina are extremely sensitive during coition and go into spasm preventing the act. She suffers from albuminous leucorrhoea mostly in the daytime without any sensation. Recurrent infections cause threatened abortion, habitual abortions.

Platina is hot patient. She has feeling of intense heat. But at the same time there is coldness and numbness in parts. While sleeping, she keeps her legs apart. Weariness is felt in the extremities. Colic in umbilical region. Sense of constriction in stomach, head and limbs. Parts are hypersensitive. Sticky stools. Intense vaginitis with pruritus vulvae.

Platina lady has strange impulses to kill somebody. She dominates others and feels herself superior to everybody. These mental disturbances are secondary to fright, grief or suppression of mental activities. Hysterical behaviour. Due to this she suffers from diseases like sterility.

MODALITIES :

< By sitting and standing, in the evening

> By walking in open air.

8.13.5 FERRUM PHOSPHORICUM

Patients requiring this drug are prone to abort repeatedly due to severe megaloblastic anaemia. Anaemia due to profuse haemorrhages. She has aversion to coition or desire is much reduced. She has marked leucorrhoea which usually starts before menses. It is thin and milky white. Patient is pale and chlorotic due to decreased iron concentration. The process of menstruation is hampered. She complains of amenorrhoea. Menses appear once in three to four months. Menstrual flow is bright red and dark. Bleeding lasts for long time. Intermittent bleeding. Irregular, late and painful periods. Membranous dysmenorrhoea with fever. There is bearing down, dull pain in the ovarian region. The supports of the uterus are relaxed, thus prolapse of uterus causing infertility. Vagina is dry and hot . This develops dyspareunia. History of gonorrhoea with heat in urethra. Gleety discharges from urethra. Burning in urethra during flow of urine. This infection spreads to the genital tract.

These ladies have oxygenoid constitution. She gets repeated attacks of fever and inflammation in various places, wasting of the muscles with emaciation. She is prone to violent local congestion of ovaries, uterus, tubes, vagina and cervix. This prevents the conception. Due to chronic gastritis she vomits off and on the undigested food material. Recurrent attacks of peritonitis and irregular menses due to recurrent inflammatory processes. Unovulatory cycles.

This remedy has marked anger. Great violence. This violence produces weakness, headache and trembling. Anxiety at night. She is unable to concentrate.

MODALITIES :

< At night (4-6 a.m.), jar, movement.

> Cold application.

8.13.6 SEPIA

Sepia has peculiar tendency to produce induration all over the genital tract. She has also marked catarrhal conditions. These form the basic ground for recurrent or chronic infections of genitourinary tract. Marked outgrowths in the cervix and in the uterus. This hampers the formation of secretory endometrium for fertilised ovum. Pelvic organs are relaxed, thus she has constant sense of bearing down as if something is protruding from the genital tract. To prevent this she develops a habit to cross her legs while sitting, lying down and even when asleep. Whenever a case of sterility comes in the consulting room and sits with her legs crossed a wise physician closes his eyes and perscribes Sepia. She has too late and scanty menses which are also irregular. There are sharp clutching pains in the vagina which radiate upwards to the uterus and then to umbilical region. Severe pains in the vagina during act of coition. Leucorrhoea is marked with intense itching, which is yellow or greenish. Male type of pelvis in females.

Portal congestion causes adverse effects on various systems, central nervous system is poorly developed. The hormones secreted by anterior pituitary are deminished so functions of genital organs are not carried out properly.

Recurrent attacks of headache secondary to hepatic disturbances. Nausea at smell and sight of food, salty taste in mouth, thus disposition to vomit after eating, white tongue, thickly coated but clean during menses. Pelvic organs are relaxed. Congestion of venous plexus in pelvic organs causes excessive vaginal secretion which is yellow, but when gets infected turns to green. This secretion probably acts as a spermicidal agent.

Sepia lady is indifferent to whom she loved best. Very irritable and easily offended. Dreads to be alone. Sad and despondent. Weeping disposition. Cannot narrate her symptoms without weeping.

MODALITIES :

< In evening, forenoon, after washing, laundry work, damp wet weather, cold air.

> Pressure, warmth of bed, hot application.

8.13.7 AGNUS CASTUS

Vagina is much relaxed due to weakness of the musculature of the vaginal walls. There is prolapse of the uterus in the introitus. Conception is prevented due to copious, thick, like white of an egg leucorrhoea. Majority of times she is infected with gonorrhoea by her partner. The sexual organs are relaxed and cold. Flabby muscles everywhere in the body. She is anaemic. Due to recurrent infections cervical, axillary and mesenteric nodes are enlarged. Profuse uterine haemorrhage when menses occur. But menses are usually suppressed. Agnus castus lady presents look of old sufferer and broken down from secret vice.

This remedy acts best in the conditions where sexual vitality is affected. There is decreased sexual ability in the patient. There is premature old age. Abuse of sexual acts. History of recurrent attacks of sexually transmitted diseases. Menses are scanty. Relaxation of genitals with leucorrhoea. Leucorrhoea is thin, transparent and yellowish which stains the clothings.

She has hysterical behaviour. Palpitation. Sexual melancholy. Fear of death. She thinks that she is sinking steadily. Forgetful, lack of courage. Mentally depressed.

Other useful remedies for sterility are

1. GOSSYPIUM
2. GRAPHITES
3. BUFO
4. SABAL SERRULATA
5. IODUM

****

TOPIC 14

TOXAEMIA OF PREGNANCY

Toxaemia of pregnancy is the condition associated with three main symptoms —

1) Hypertension

2) Oedema and

3) Proteinuria and other hronic renal diseases.

Previously it was claimed that toxic substances are found in blood during pregnancy. But later on it was proved that no such toxic substances were traceable in this condition. Thus at present these symptoms are described as "pre-eclampsia" and "eclampsia". Pre-eclampsia is the syndrome having -

1) High blood pressure ranging between 140-160 (systolic) and 90-100 (diastolic) mm of Hg.

2) Oedema of pitting type and

3) Proteinuria.

When pre-eclampsia is complicated with convulsion, patient goes into eclampsia condition.

8.14.1 CICUTA VIROSA

Vertigo with gastralgia. Head turned or twisted to one side. Cerebrospinal irritation. The head is drawn back. Patient takes opisthotonous position. The limbs are rigid and convulsed. She has strange desire to eat coal and many other such things. She is full of vertigo. Things turn around in a circle. Vertigo on walking, glassy eyes. Semilateral headache forcing the patient to sit. Headache as if the brain would loosen on walking. First there is spasm in the head, then it descends.

Head is hot and the limbs are cold. Head or scalp is covered with cold sweat at night. Spasms or cramps in the muscles of nape of neck. Pupils are dilated. Strabismus. Convulsions are induced by slight touch, motion, jar and cold.

Sensation of coldness in heart. All complaints spread from heart or chest. Nose is sensitive to touch. Jar and noise bring complaints. All complaints are associated with hypersensitivity. Skin shows various skin eruptions.

Peevishness, delirium and stupid feeling. She is indifferent. Moaning or crying. Melancholic lady.

MODALITIES :

< Draughts of air, tobacco, smoke, touch.

8.14.2 CUPRUM METALLICUM

Tonic convulsions in late months of pregnancy call for this remedy. In these patients the thumb is affected first. Thumb is drawn into palm and rest of the fingers are clenched around it. Tonic contractions of limbs. Limbs are drawn upward with great violence. Jerking and twitching movements of legs. Many times this state of convulsions terminate in a state of stasis, when the functions of mind are diminished. Convulsions after whooping cough. Cuprum patient has cramps in each and every muscle of the body-legs, hands, and so on. The patient suddenly becomes blind. Sensation as if all lights have disappeared from the room. Labour pains cease and convulsions sets in. Convulsion start from fingers or toes or from lower part of chest and then spread to all the muscles. Blueness and coldness of the limbs, toes, fingers and nails. Convulsions from suppression of discharges. Spasmodic closing of eyelids, rotates the eyeball suddenly. Nausea, vomiting and diarrhoea associated with the spasms. She feels pressure on the stomach. Congestion of head. Uraemic convulsions. Pulse is hard, full and quick with palpitation. Convulsions with suppressed and scanty urine. Violent vomiting, she has hysterical attitude. This hysterical attitude may change into St. Vitus' dance. Tingling sensation in the head with hypertension.

Periodical complaints and these start on left side. Chorea is from fright. Cholera morbus. Whooping cough with three successive attacks and it is spasmodic, makes her cyanosed. Cough is relieved by drinking cold water. Cough may bring on vomiting of food. Convulsions from cough. Taking out and in of the tongue. Skin is bluish and itching in spots. Sleep is more and deep. There is rumbling in abdomen.

MODALITIES :

< Least touch, vomiting, cough, night.

> By sweating, taking cold water.

8.14.3 GLONOINE

Excessive blood flow to the head and heart. Tremendous pulsations all over the body. The mouth and eyelids are dry. Face is red. Confused state of mind with loss of conciousness. Sudden congesion of the head and severe headache starts. She wants the head high and cold applications over it. Convulsions during pregnancy with severe headache and dimness of vision. She has typical behaviour during pregnancy. Headache is so severe that she wants to jump from the window. Headache starts from the occipital region and goes to the forehead. Every motion is so painful that the Glonoine patient remains in the same position for hours together. The lady is constipated. Oedema of the extremities; and also of the abdominal wall. Strenuous breathing; as if control over breathing is lost. Intense hot, burning sensation on vertex. Burning, hot sensation in nape of neck and between the scapular regions. Flushed face but if patient is aggravated, face becomes dusky in appearance.

All the troubles are due to exposure to bright light or heat of oven, sun etc. or after fear, fright etc. Dyspnoea, fluttering of the heart. Pulsations all over the body. Congestion of head with dizziness. Head feels too large. Headache increases with heat of sun and declines with decrease in the heat. She has feeling of fullness of neck. Aching of face with flushing, then perspiration. Hyperaesthesia of neck and upper part of back.

Fainting spells with cerebral congestion. Swelling of neck, ears, throat chokes her and she keeps them uncovered.

Mentally she has confusion and irritability. Great weariness of mind and body. She has no desire for work. Least contradiction exites her.

MODALITIES :

< Heat of sun, stooping, jar, stimulants, rest.

> Cold air, cold application, brandy.

8.14.4 APIS MELLIFICA

Apis is a very good remedy to treat toxaemia of pregnancy if the generalities and mental picture allow. It has all the symptoms of toxaemia. Firstly this remedy shows inflammation and hyperaemia of every system and parts. Parts are red, hot and painful. Oedema both local and generalised. Oedema is widespread in the body. Puffy bag-like swellings are seen. Swollen lower eyelids. Dropsy of lower extremities and face. Oedema extends to submucous layer. It establishes serous effusions in the parts. Dropsy, catarrh and erysipelas are found in Apis. In all these dropsical conditions there are stinging and burning pains. She has thick rash all over the body. Pitting type of oedema. Notable general anasarca. Swollen face. Greatly thickened abdominal wall. Mucous membranes of the body seem to discharge water on pinching. This dropsical condition is many times associated with cardiac congestion. High blood pressure with angina. This is a good remedy for fits in pregnancy due to toxaemia. Urine is scanty, comes only in drops. She has to strain much before passing urine. After these efforts she could void little quantity of urine. Intense burning of urethra during urination. Urine is loaded with albumin. Nephritis, urethritis, with albuminuria mark this remedy. Many times there is inflammation of the uterus and ovaries and dreadful oedema over the external genitalia. All these may result in stillbirth but Apis not only prevents stillbirth but also helps to induce normal labour.

Apis is known for oedema and typical stinging and burning pains. Very much prostrated lady. Sense of constrictions everywhere in the body and so she wants to remove all the clothings from the body especially around the abdomen. She feels very drowsy and likes to sleep all the time but she is aggravated after sleep. Dyspnoea, suffocative feeling due to oedema of larynx. Soreness of skin. Fiery red and oedematous tongue. Photophobia with sharp pains. Suppuration of eyes.

Stupor, sudden cries, very awkward, nervous and irritable lady. Tearful mood.

MODALITIES :

< Heat in general, touch, closed room, after sleep.

> Cold open air, uncovering.

8.14.5 GELSEMIUM

The heart is feeble and the pulse is soft, feeble and irregular. Lady complains of palpitation off and on. Cerebral hyperaemia. Excessive blood flow to brain or spinal cord. Eyes are congested and pupils are dilated. Lachrymation and twitching of eyelids. Patient feels dazed. Diplopia with dimness of vision. The vision appears full of dark spots. Drooping of eyelids. Great heaviness of the limbs. Patient feels weak and exhausted. Tearing sensation felt in nerves all over the body due to inflammatory condition. There is coldness running up the back from the sacral region. The headache is so violent that the patient cannot stand and lies down as if paralysed from pains. Neuralgic pains with nausea and vomiting. Nervous excitement, this is usually from fear and embassment and shock. Paralytic condition of the sphincter. Involuntary loss of stools and urine. Loss of sensation in the parts. During febrile conditions, she has profound sleep and coma.

All the complaints of Gelsemium lady are attended with dullness, dizziness and drowsiness and trembling of whole body. Coryza is always associated with fever and headache. Headache is relieved by profuse urination. Oppression of chest and great weakness cause slowness of respiration. Spasm of glottis may lead to attack of dyspnoea. Various skin eruptions with livid spots and skin is dry and hot. She has weak, slow pulse with palpitation and she fears that her heart will stop beating if she stops moving. Tonsillitis with shooting pains extending to ear. Chilliness is marked.

Mentally the lady is very dull and lethargic. Wants to be left alone and she has absolute lack of fear. Nervous diarrhoea. Apathetic to everything and her illness too. Easily excitable.

MODALITIES :

< Heat and rest in geneal, dampness, excitement.

> Motion, profuse urination, open air.

8.14.6 BELLADONNA

Great sensitivity with throbbing headache. Shooting pains in temporal region due to congestion of head. Patient rolls head from side to side on pillow. Inflammatory condition of eyes with objects glistening. Pupils are dilated. Redness with burning. Dimness of vision with actual blindness in toxaemia of pregnancy. There is great dryness of the oral cavity, eyes, nostrils etc. Vertigo with intense excitability. Turning in bed or moving the head makes her dizzy. Things go round. Vertigo with pulsations of every larger arteries. She is hypersensitive and craves sympathy. Spasms, general or local. Group of muscles goes in spasm. Tonic and clonic spasms. Burning in throat with inflammation of tonsillar glands. Inflammation of uterine mucous membrane, ovaries and tubes. Retention of urine due to recurrent urinary tract infection.

Urine is turbid and scanty, associated with tenesmus. Incontinence of urine and complaints of frequent micturition of profuse quantity. During eclamptic condition she has a sense of pressure on the pelvic organs. Sensation as if all the viscera would protrude through vagina. Violent palpitation. Pulse is rapid but weak. Shooting pains along the knees with jerking. She has very restless sleep. Pain and sense of fullness especially in forehead.

Congestion of every organ with heat, redness and dryness is marked in Belladonna. Skin is dry and hot. Glands are inflamed. Convulsive motion of facial muscles and she is very sleepless but feels drowsy all the time. Restlessness is also marked. Hyper-sensitive to noise, photopnobia. Autophony. Swollen, red, painful and hot joints. Neuralgic pains. Hyperaesthesia of body. Mouth and throat are very dry and she has thirst for cold water but she has dread of drinking due to vomiting. Dysphagia. Throbbing of every vessel in the body. Exertion brings on palpitation and laborious breathing.

Mentally she is very violent and she has visual hallucinations. Delirium with red face and congestion of head. She bites and strikes people. She uses absurd language. Violent insanity, unconsciousness.

MODALITIES :

< Any external stimulus, night, uncovering the head, touch, jar and motion, draught of air, heat of sun.

> In warm room, semi-erect position, rest.

Other important remedies for toxaemia of pregnancy are

1. MERC. CORROSIVUS
2. ZINCUM METALLICUM
3. MEDORRHINUM
4. SAMBUCUS NIGRA
5. BARYTA MUR.

****

REFERENCES

1.	Handbook of Materia Medica & Homoeopathic Therapeutics	T.F. Allen
2.	Materia Medica Pura	Hahnemann
3.	Repertory of Homoeopahtic Materia Medica	J.T. Kent
4.	Textbook of Pathology	William Boyd
5.	The encyclopedia of Pure Materia Medica	T.F. Allen
6.	Clinical Materia Medica	E.A. Farrington
7.	Lectures on Materia Medica	Carroll Dunham
8.	Principles of Surgery	Seymour I. Schwartz
9.	Textbook of obstetrics & Neonatology	Dawn
10.	Textbook of Gynaecology	Shaw
11.	Materia Medica with Repertory	Boericke
12.	Boenninghausen's Characteristics & Repertory	C.M. Boger
13.	Clinical Surgery	S. Das
14.	Homoeopathic Drug Pictures	M.L. Tyler
15.	Comparative Materia Medica	E.A. Farrington
16.	Pathology Illustrated	A.D.T. Govan P.A. Macfarlane R. Callonder
17.	Lectures on Homoeopathic Materia Medica	J.T. Kent